BORROWED TIME

Living with Cancer with Someone you Love

FRED EDGE

Borrowed Time

Living with Cancer
with Someone you Love

oolichan books
LANTZVILLE, BRITISH COLUMBIA, CANADA
1995

Canadian Cataloguing in Publication Data

Edge, Fred, 1927-
Borrowed time

Includes bibliographical references and index.

ISBN 0-88982-148-8

1. Cancer—Patients—Home care. 2. Cancer—Patients—Family relationships. 3. Cancer—Treatment—Popular works.
I. Title.
RC262.E33 1995   362.1'96994   C95-910248-5

Quotation on page 82 from *The Poetry of Robert Frost* edited by Edward Connery Lathem. Copyright 1951 by Robert Frost. Copyright 1923 © 1969 by Henry Holt and Co., Inc. Reprinted by permission of Henry Holt and Co., Inc.

The publisher gratefully acknowledges the assistance of the Canada Council.

Published by
Oolichan Books
P.O. Box 10
Lantzville, British Columbia
Canada, V0R 2H0

Printed in Canada by
Hignell Printing Limited
Winnipeg, Manitoba

*To those with cancer
and those who love them.
From Chris*

Contents

· Author's Note

Borrowed Time is not a medical book.

It neither recommends nor rejects conventional medical procedures. Nor does it dismiss alternative treatment, while at the same time not subscribing to the notion of the "miracle cure."

It is one couple's personal journey, over eight years, through the peaks and valleys of living with cancer: what my wife and I learned about it and how we learned to cope with it.

It is important that you realize that you and your spouse— or your mother, father, sister or brother—are not alone. There are hundreds of thousands of other couples and families who have the same wrenching medical problem you have. Accepting this and understanding the disease is your first step towards learning how to deal with it, with as little trauma and as successfully as possible.

My wife and I were what you might call an average couple, if there is any such thing. You couldn't say our marriage was made in heaven. You couldn't say it was made in hell. Like most marriages that last, I think it was made somewhere in-between.

We were both strong-willed, volatile people, pursuing separate careers and periodically, because of this, separate lives. The glue that held us together over the jarring times, and there were a few of these over the years, was the love that had brought us together in the first place. When we learned that Chris had cancer, that bond became even stronger.

At some point during that period, I saw an interview on television with some American celebrity or other. His name is not worth remembering. He said that when he and his wife found out she had cancer, he had left her. He explained, "I just couldn't hack it."

Sitting alone in the living-room, I felt an overwhelming sadness for this woman. Her husband had performed the ultimate act of selfishness. Because of this, at the most difficult time of her life, she had suffered the ultimate desertion. I wish I could have gone to her and held her hand. Instead, I went to my wife, who was reading and resting in the bedroom, and held hers.

I just wish there had been a *Borrowed Time* out there for us. We could have avoided so much trial and error; so much of having to learn the hard way.

Chris did extensive research and kept detailed diaries towards this book. She made me promise to write it. She intended to provide laypersons like ourselves with a plainly written, better understanding of cancer. She also wanted *Borrowed Time* to suggest ways to handle it, both personally and within the family.

Finally, most importantly, she wanted to say this:

Listen to all the professional advice.

Ask questions and learn all you can about your condition.

Then decide for yourself how you wish to deal with it.

It is your life.

"Living well is the best revenge."

Foreign proverb translated by George Herbert (1593-1633)

1 · When cancer struck

My wife, Chris, had been told she had a tumor.

Was it malignant?

We shared the cautious reply in her doctor's office: "Not necessarily."

I glanced at my wife and saw from her expression that she was thinking the same thing I was.

My God, didn't they have some way of knowing? They weren't sure whether her condition was a dirty word or a clean one, malignant or benign.

They would not know for sure, the doctor explained, until they operated, took a slice of tissue, and had the hospital lab do a biopsy. If the tumor proved cancerous, time was critical. Chris was scheduled for major surgery the following Monday to have it removed.

I drove her to the hospital a couple of days later. It was just before noon on a Saturday that we left our home in Winnipeg's River Heights for the short drive to the Misericordia.

The Misericordia is a Catholic teaching hospital with an affectionate alias: The Misery. Right now, I knew my wife wasn't feeling all that friendly towards it. "I was born in that hospital," she had said the night before, with a wry try at humor. "I don't want to die there!"

We chose to drive the roundabout way, "the scenic route" Chris always enjoyed, past the park-like grounds and palatial homes on Wellington Crescent.

She was looking at them, but I felt she wasn't really seeing them.

"Did the doctors tell you anything?"

It was a question she had asked me more than once over the past while.

I learned early that the possibility that you have cancer breeds paranoia. You begin to wonder if your doctors, friends, even your own family, are keeping things from you. Chris was no exception.

I gave her my usual answer. "Nothing they haven't told you."

I realized that I didn't sound too convincing.

"I told McIntyre, Rogers, and the other guy, the surgeon—Broder—what you've said from the start: You want it all up front. No lies. No kid gloves. Everything straight."

She almost smiled. "I sound so damned brave," she said. "I'm scared to death!"

I took one hand off the wheel and used it to cover the clenched fist on the seat between us.

"What if I have colon cancer?" Chris said. "Dear God in heaven!"

We were early. Check-in time wasn't for another hour or so. We decided to stay on Wellington Crescent, past the bridge over the Red River that borders the hospital, and have lunch at an Osborne Village café called The Courtyard. Chris said she wasn't all that hungry, but for at least a while longer she would not have to commit herself to The Misery.

We parked on the other side of an intersection that was a few doors up from the café. Our spur-of-the-moment lunch date had lifted our spirits. Like a couple of schoolkids playing hookey, we clasped hands and ran the light. We must have looked like we didn't have a care in the world!

The maitre d' showed us to a table for two overlooking the Village.

We both had a martini, dry with a lemon twist, a rare choice for Chris so early in the day. We ordered a variation of *escalope de veau*. Looking out over the traffic on Osborne, I remembered it had been a favorite entrée at a family café called *La Bonne Table* when we were first married and living in Paris. There had been few problems then. Certainly none like the one we faced now.

The Courtyard's version of the veal dish was filleted breast of chicken. It was served with crusty chunks of French bread to sop up the well-remembered cream and mushroom sauce. We shared a bottle of our favorite California wine, a Robert Mondavi *fumé blanc*.

Martinis and wine are not the smartest way to self-prep for entry into hospital. Particularly when you've been diagnosed as possibly suffering from colon cancer. Chris said she didn't care. She had been a healthy, privileged, and generally happy person all her life. She had been hospitalized on only three previous occasions. These had been to give birth to our three sons, Rory, Casey, and Shawn, at Women's College Hospital in Toronto.

Confronted with the spectre of cancer since our visit to the doctor's office, she felt betrayed. How and why, she had wondered aloud, can this be happening?

"Other people get cancer. Other people die from it. Not me."

We had no way of knowing on that drive to The Misery, eight years before what Chris came to call her "borrowed time" ran out, that this was just the beginning.

Within a few days, her surgeon, Dr. Morris Broder, removed a large tumor in a procedure called a sigmoid colon resection. It proved to be malignant. Three years later, she underwent emergency surgery for ovarian cancer, the same type that took the life of actress and television comedian Gilda Radner. This was followed by four sessions, over sixteen weeks, of in-hospital chemotherapy.

Eighteen months later, in October, 1988, doctors found that a "pelvic mass" was obstructing her bowel. They decided it was too risky at this time for her to undergo a third critical operation. She had barely survived the last one.

Radiation to shrink this obstruction, taken at Calgary's Tom Baker Cancer Centre, led to the discovery that a "beauty mark" on her right shoulder had turned ugly. Diagnosed as melanoma, a potentially fatal skin cancer, the malignant mole and a section of the tissue surrounding it were removed surgically.

Early in 1990, Chris would undergo further tests and major surgery at two Toronto hospitals, Mount Sinai and Toronto General.

Throughout all this, which included twice being told by doctors that she was "terminal," we would both learn a great deal about coexisting with cancer. My wife would learn to ask questions and what questions to ask. She would learn to expect answers; to demand them, when necessary. Faced with three malignancies, each one a potential killer, she would learn to make the decisions that would have a direct bearing on whether she lived or died.

"In either case," she said, "I will have the satisfaction of knowing that whatever happens to me will be the result of my own choices, not someone else's."

There were two important results from this period in our lives. One was that Chris learned to be responsible both to and for herself. The other was the discovery that if you work hard enough at it, there are two self-administered "miracle drugs" that can keep you alive. One is a positive attitude with, as surprising as this may sound, a good sense of humor. The other is the understanding and supportiveness of the person who shares your love and your life.

Colon cancer is not easily diagnosed. It is not something that a woman can self-examine for in the shower, as she can for the lumps that suggest the possibility of breast cancer. My wife's own small warning signal hardly seemed worth getting excited about. Over a period of several months, she had become chronically constipated.

Our family physician, Dr. Donald McIntyre, was recovering from a severe case of respiratory arrest. Chris saw his substitute. After a brief interrogation and a digital rectal examination, he said that she showed signs of "lazy bowel syndrome." He advised her to increase her fibre intake by eating a bran cereal for breakfast and to spend more time sitting on the toilet. In case this didn't work, he prescribed Senokot, a gentle laxative that he assured her would "wake up" her lazy bowel.

"It's lazy, all right," Chris quipped a few weeks later, on a return visit to her doctor. "Like in Rip van Winkle!"

He scheduled her for a barium enema and picture-taking session with X-rays.

For twenty-four hours prior to this procedure, your diet consists of nothing by Jello, consommé, and clear liquids. You also dose with castor oil and self-administer a suppository laxative the night before. Cut-off time for everything, including water, is midnight.

I shared my wife's breakfast, luncheon, and dinner of consommé and Jello with the lame excuse that it presented a good opportunity to lose a pound or two. She accused me of being chivalrous. I was too hungry to argue with her. Later, while we were watching Knowlton Nash do the CBC-TV National at ten o'clock, I poured myself a Ballantyne's and water. Chris asked if I thought Scotch qualified as a "clear fluid." I considered the similarity in appearance between Scotch and consommé and said I didn't see why not.

Chris said later that she must have been spaced out on Jello and concern over what the next morning might bring. She had two drinks. While we never knew for sure, she figured that those few ounces of Scotch might have helped blow the next day's tests right out of the water.

She said that if she had known that evening what she learned the next morning, she wouldn't have done anything even remotely likely to jeopardize them.

"It just isn't worth it, to have to go through all that all over again."

My wife's X-rays were taken in the radiology room of the Medical Arts building. For this procedure, the patient lies on one side, strapped to a table-top that tilts at the operator's touch of a lever. A tube is inserted into the rectum. The barium enema, a chalky white liquid, is pumped into the bowel. While the table-top is tipped every which way, an X-ray camera shoots pictures. Barium sulphate is a metallic chemical. It reveals the intestine in silhouette, highlighting whatever and wherever the problem is.

From start to finish, the photo session took about an hour. I had been sitting, thumbing through old copies of *Macleans* magazine and *Readers Digest*, in the reception room. The X-ray technician's assistant steered Chris past me into the john. My wife was wearing one of those white sheets slit down the back. She made a face that plainly said she wasn't having fun.

After about fifteen minutes, the technician's assistant came back and told Chris she could get dressed. The idea is to make sure the bowel has emptied itself of barium before you leave.

We had agreed to celebrate the end of our fast by having brunch at Oscar's, a popular downtown deli not far from the Medical Arts. We both ordered coffee and bagels with lox and cream cheese, a house specialty. About halfway home, it abruptly became obvious that the technician's assistant had miscalculated and that a bowel given a barium cocktail, as Chris ruefully put it, loses all sense of propriety. One moment she said she was feeling a little tired, looking forward to getting home after the ordeal of the morning. The next her clothes and the passenger seat of our Ford Thunderbird were a mess.

After all that, the tests proved inconclusive. Something, perhaps helped along by the Scotch late the night before, had clouded the results. My wife's stand-in physician offered to reschedule the tests. Chris refused. "No way am I going to go through that all over again," she said. "Not so soon." Not when the fasting and physical distress were still fresh in her mind.

Besides, her condition seemed not nearly as bad as it had been. She was taking reasonably good care of herself. We both recently had gone cold turkey on cigarettes after years of smoking a couple of cartons a week. We were dong what Chris called "jalking" (walking and jogging) three miles or so every morning along the dirt path and pleasantly treed median that runs much of the length of Wellington Crescent.

My wife had always agreed with the late Duchess of Windsor that you can never be too rich or too thin. Rich was unlikely. Thin she was working on, striving to drop about ten pounds through our daily "jalks" and cutting back on rich foods and starches. Given her common-sense weight loss program and a high-fibre diet, she decided that whatever her condition was, she could live with it.

She was wrong. Within three months, her symptoms became more pronounced. The problem, as it turned out, was that they weren't all that conclusive. She had experienced a change in bowel pattern, which could be caused by any number of things. Sometimes now her movements were pencil-thin, but there was neither blood-spotting nor excessive flatulence, which are more clearly signs of colon cancer. She was having a random pain in her lower right side that struck without warning. She described it as a brief, stabbing stitch, so severe that it sometimes made her gasp.

Our family doctor was seeing patients again. Through sheer determination and extensive physical therapy, Dr. McIntyre had recovered remarkably from the crippling effects of the respiratory arrest he had suffered. He scheduled Chris for a simple X-ray of the lower abdomen and pelvic region.

"I think there might be something there," he advised. "Let's get a better look."

On our way out of Dr. McIntyre's office, Chris groaned her displeasure. "Barium enema time again!" she said, but her protest was to me, not Dr. McIntyre. We both had a lot of confidence in this man. He is one of the "Old School" of general practitioners who still make house calls, and a fine diagnostician. He also is a Renaissance Man who can discuss knowledgeably just about everything under the sun. I have often wished that Dr. McIntyre had been there for my wife from the beginning, rather than the substitute who had sat in for him while he was recovering.

This time, Chris and I both made sure she did everything right. She said she also had a more skilful practitioner who had made the procedure less painful. When it was all over, she sat on the john for twice as long as she had the first time. When the technician's assistant came for her after what she thought was time enough, Chris waved her away.

She was learning, and she was teaching me in the process. When you decide to be primarily responsible for your own well-being, to take your life in your own hands, it soon becomes clear that not all doctors, nurses, and medical technicians are created equal. They would like us to believe they are, that we and those we love are all somehow safe under the umbrella of their professional mystique, but this is simply not so. Medical personnel, like plumbers and automobile mechanics, come with varying degrees of commitment and competence. They range from the inspired to the mediocre to the shockingly inept. They can be dedicated or casual, caring or negligent. The confusion for the patient lies in the fact that their office walls are all basically hung with the same credentials.

We had an appointment with Dr. McIntyre, on the eighth floor of the Medical Arts building, on the same day that he saw her barium X-rays. His reaction to them was as cautious as it had been to the previous ones.

"There's something there," he said, frowning, "but I still don't know what it is."

It was clear, however, that something was obstructing the

bowel. To this day, I don't know why Chris and I remained almost unconcerned. Possibly it was because we both assumed she had diverticulitis, a condition she thought she might have inherited. Her father had had a diverticulum, the medical term for an abnormal, pouch-like balloon, on the wall of the colon. Not considered terribly serious, it had been removed surgically. While Chris and I stood around, admiring the modern art hung in Dr. McIntyre's office, he got on the phone and pressed for an early appointment with an internist.

That was another of the things that Chris and I liked about our family doctor. When he decided what had to be done, whether it was treating you himself or bringing in a specialist, it was done right then. In his care, you felt not only in competent hands, but special, like you were the only patient in the world. I think to Don McIntyre's way of thinking, you were.

As the title implies, Dr. Arnold Rogers is a specialist in internal disorders and diseases. His office is just around the corner from the Medical Arts in an aging block called The Doctors Building. You can climb a broad flight of stairs to the common waiting-room with small, flanking offices on the second floor, or you can ride a tired old elevator. We took the stairs.

Chris sat and thumbed through a magazine. All around us sat very glum-looking people; very sick-looking people. With them were other people, like me, who were doing their best to look reassuring. I privately hoped that Arnold Rogers was more impressive than his surroundings.

Chris must have read my mind. "Anybody this busy," she said, "has to be good."

Dr. Rogers and his receptionist use a revolving door system to process patients. While one is being interviewed or examined in one of the two cubbyholes off the crowded waiting-room, another is waiting in the second.

The receptionist called out "Mrs. Edge." We entered the small room together, closing the door behind us. At my wife's request, we had begun doing these interviews in partnership. This not only provided Chris with moral support, but gave me a better understanding of the problem and how I might help her cope with it. This was especially important when we finally learned how serious her situation was.

We could hear Dr. Rogers' deep voice and frequent laughter on the other side of the wall. We were to learn that wherever he goes, this cheerfully noisy space goes with him. It fills offices and hospital rooms and corridors. Like the lunch that sits on his desk, which he brown-bags from home, and the ill-fitting clothes that give him the look of a rumpled bear, it is part of his "schtick."

He entered the room and introduced himself. He talked a while with Chris about her medical problems, past and present. He had already studied the barium X-rays. He explained the next procedure. Then he opened the door and called out to his receptionist to set up an appointment at The Misery. Chris was given instructions for a self-prep, which was pretty much the same as the one for the barium X-rays.

"It's fun-time again," she said, as we took the stairs down to the street. She didn't have to elaborate: Jello, consommé, laxatives, and suppositories.

Little did we know.

As Chris said later, it is one thing to have liquid chalk pumped into your rectum through a rubber tube. It's quite another to be draped over a barrel-like table while someone carries out an in-depth examination with a sigmoidoscope.

This is a rod, preferably the flexible fiberoptic type, with a light at one end. It serves as a sort of periscope.

She was given a Valium to help her relax. Dr. Rogers tried to be gentle. He used the stock phrase doctors use when something is really going to hurt: This may be a little unpleasant.

"It was extremely unpleasant," Chris said.

She did not, however, find it humiliating, as some patients do. My wife never thought to play what she called "mind-games" with medical procedures that might help keep her alive.

During the procedure, Dr. Rogers did a biopsy. He took snippets from a small polyp, or tumor, that had grown on the mucous wall of her intestine, as well as from the wall itself. These were sent to the lab for analysis. When it was all over, the nurse guided her into another room and told her to lie down and rest a while. Chris said that after about fifteen minutes, she felt able to go.

She said the nurse seemed a little surprised. "Are you sure?"

"Positive."

My wife never liked hospitals.

I was waiting for her in the sitting-room between Emergency and Oncology. Despite the fact that she told me she felt okay, as she had the nurse, I thought she looked a little shaky.

"How was it?" I asked.

"It could have been worse; but not much."

I squeezed her arm.

A few days later we returned to the Doctors Building. Dr. Rogers had received the results from the biopsy. He joked around with one of those "good news-bad news" routines that hadn't yet become trite.

"I have good news and bad," he said. "The good news is that your tumor is benign."

Chris and I exchanged a quick look. Our happy hearts did a somersault in tandem.

"The bad news is that I'm still suspicious."

He waited for this to sink in. I remember that neither of us let it. Drowning people don't throw back lifelines.

"I'd like to do it one more time," he said. "Just to be sure."

My wife's expression told me that was okay with her. Just about anything, including what she later laughed off as "another merry waltz with the sigmoidoscope," was okay with her. Her tumor had checked out benign. That was all she needed or wanted to know.

This time, and in times yet to come, she did it without Valium. Chris was one of those people who had both a high drug tolerance and a high pain threshold. This meant that relaxants like Valium and pain-killers like Demerol, administered in like amounts, didn't do as much for her as they do for most people. At the same time, she could cope with levels of pain that others might find intolerable. I don't know whether this was good or bad. It's just the way it was.

The big problem when you have a high tolerance for both drugs and pain is this: when the pain gets so bad that you really do need something to control it, a normal dose of drugs won't do. This is a problem Chris would suffer for quite some time, until the doctors close to her came to understand it. With those who didn't, she eventually learned to take her own precautions.

Our minds have a way of blocking out those things we don't want to remember. This is how it was with Chris on that morning in March, 1984, in Dr. Rogers' office, when we learned she had cancer.

She didn't recall him telling us the second biopsy had revealed a malignancy and that he was arranging for surgery the following week. She did not remember smiling politely and responding: "Thank you for all your help, Doctor."

Thank you for telling me I have cancer.

It was on our walk through the sitting-room to the stairs that her mind dropped its guard and her memory kicked in. "I have to have an operation," she said, as though we both hadn't just heard this. "I have a malignancy."

At that point, she couldn't bring herself to say the word cancer.

We descended the stairs to the street and stood outside the entrance to the building. All around us, people without cancer hurried by on their way to lunch, or shopping. Or on some errand or other. As devastating as the disease itself are the fear and feeling of helplessness it generates. For thirty-four years, Chris had been my best friend, as well as my wife. She looked afraid and confused. I took her arm and squeezed it. "Let's go home," I said. It occurred to me that I was squeezing her arm a lot lately. We walked in silence to where I had parked the car.

Chris always prided herself on her sense of orderliness. Once, some years ago, when she and I and the three children had leased a yacht for the weekend and were cruising on Lake Simcoe, north of Toronto, we struck an unmarked rock. The breached hull began taking on buckets of water.

In the overall confusion, I heard my wife call out to the kids: "Strip the bunks and fold your bedding!"

That's the way she was. If we were going to sink, by golly, we were going to sink neat!

As it turned out, I was able to head the boat for shore and run it aground in shallow water before we foundered.

Chris carried this same sense of "sinking neat" with her on her many hospital stays over the next eight years. Establishing and maintaining an unshakeable sense of self, together with a reasonable level of personal comfort, did not come easily. This was her first voyage of discovery into the shadowy world of oncology, the word, rooted in Greek, for the study and treatment of tumors. She was setting sail with as much blind faith and as little actual knowledge as Christopher Columbus had.

When we got home, she phoned Mario, her hairdresser. He and his staff usually work on a one-week appointment schedule. When she told him she was entering hospital on the weekend, he magically found time for her the next morning. Then she phoned Bev, who did her manicures and pedicures, and had no trouble getting booked for Friday.

Chris told me when I came for her that both Mario and Bev had expressed regret that she was being hospitalized and hoped that it was nothing serious. She said she had thanked them and changed the subject. She was not yet ready to talk about it. She was not yet ready to say, "Yes, well, I've got cancer."

We both noticed that people, even friends and relatives, react badly when you tell them that. They begin to look at you too compassionately. Their eyes are already saying goodbye.

Chris didn't want anyone's pity. Besides, there was still some hope. The results of the first biopsy, done by Dr. Rogers on snippets he had taken from the small polyp on the mucous wall of her intestine, had been benign. The second had been malignant. When we asked him if this meant that the tumor in her colon was malignant, he had replied "Not necessarily."

We were hanging our hopes on that. Chris did not see any point in saying she had cancer if there was a chance that a biopsy of the actual tumor might prove otherwise. I agreed with her.

We adopted a "let's wait and see" attitude.

This was fine for the next couple of days. It was not until the evening before my wife's entry into hospital that something approaching panic set in.

Never mind the simple prospect of major surgery. Dr. Rogers had introduced us to his colleague, Morris Broder, who would perform the operation. During a digital examination, Dr. Broder had mentioned the possibility of a colostomy. If Chris had colon cancer, her chances were one in five that she would need an artificial anus cut into her abdomen. Called a stoma, it would channel bowel movements into a bag she would have to wear.

To lose that thought, she tried to keep busy. She had put together a hospital wardrobe of two pretty nightgowns, what turned out to be a completely impractical pair of designer slippers with heels, and an elegant robe. She packed these—along with her Shalimar perfume, lipstick, powder, creams, Dove soap, toothbrush, and toothpaste, makeup mirror, comb, and hairbrush—in the nylon overnighter she called her "happy bag" because of its contrasting bright colors.

While my wife packed, I went down to the corner convenience store for *Vogue*, *Vanity Fair*, and *Time Magazine*. She already had begun *Matriarch*, the best-selling royal biography by Anne Edwards.

The last item to go into the "happy bag" was a framed photo of us both, taken by a friend the previous fall at the Centre for the Arts in Banff, Alberta.

I had been a resident writer at the Leighton Artist

Colony, working on the final draft of a biography of Charlotte Ross, the first woman doctor to practise in Quebec and the Canadian West. My wife had been a journalist when we met. In the way we shared so many aspects of our married lives, we had researched the book together.

❧

It was going on two o'clock on the Saturday afternoon Chris was scheduled for the surgery that would enable Dr. Broder to do a biopsy on the tumor in her colon. We had lingered as long as we could over a third cup of coffee in the Courtyard Café. It was hospital check-in time. We drove back along Wellington Crescent and over the bridge to The Misery.

I saw my wife through Admitting and up to her room. I helped her unpack and stayed until she got settled in. I left with the promise to return that evening with a box of Kleenex, a pillow, and her mohair bed-throw. Even then, in 1986, hospitals had begun cost-cutting on such take-for-granted things as personal tissues, an additional pillow, and an extra blanket.

We were learning.

After that first surgery, Chris never entered hospital without bringing these three items with her. As her condition worsened, requiring monthly overnight stays for chemotherapy, or an emergency admittance, she also kept on hand a "hospital bag" pre-packed with bedclothes and toiletries.

Over the next forty-eight hours, Chris was "prepped" by the hospital team of orderlies, technicians, nurses, and doctors who prepare patients for surgery. Other than myself, her younger brother Don, and our youngest son, Shawn, she had no visitors who were not professionally involved. This was by choice. I wondered if she was trying to downplay the seriousness of her situation, hoping, perhaps subconsciously, that this might somehow make it go away. I knew for sure that she did not want to be an alarmist.

My wife's mother, Johan, was ninety-four years old and living in Tuxedo Villa, a Winnipeg home for seniors. Just the year before, she had lost the elder of her two sons, Charlie, to heart disease. My wife was her only daughter. Her first had died in infancy. Chris did not want her mother to know that not only was she going in for major surgery, but that it might prove she had cancer.

Our son Shawn was regularly in and out of town as the drummer in a Winnipeg-based rock band. Neither of his brothers was living here. Rory, the eldest of the three, was a lawyer with the Justice Department in Ottawa. Casey was doing grass roots public relations for the City of Calgary, working in what he called "the complaints department."

I suggested to my wife it was only fair that we phone Rory and Casey and tell them of their mother's impending surgery.

"I know you're positive that the operation will go well," I said. "So am I. But what about that chance-in-a-million that it doesn't?

It's not easy playing the guy in the black hat, especially when it's with someone you love.

"We can't keep this from the boys," I said.

We finally reached a compromise. Chris said it was okay to phone, but to tell them not to go to the trouble and expense of coming home. I was to sell them on this on the basis that the surgery was routine and her prognosis was great; there really was nothing to worry about.

After making the calls, I reported back that it had been

difficult talking Casey out of catching the next flight out of Calgary for Winnipeg. Rory had been no problem. The law is our eldest son's adoptive family. He was working on an important case.

Most of us, probably influenced by the unreality of television, picture surgeons as tall, slim, and toothy, like airline pilots. Morris Broder is a stocky man. His skilful fingers are stubby. His movements are abrupt, like his moments of humor. There was confidence, but not humor, in the brief talk the three of us had the night before he operated.

"I don't think you'll need a colostomy," he said, speaking to Chris but addressing us both, "but don't hold me to that. It depends on how much of the intestine I have to remove and how high up the tumor is."

The manicure and pedicure that Chris had gotten on the same day that Mario had done her hair had been a waste of time. She was brought a bottle of nail polish remover and a wad of absorbent cotton to wipe her fingernails and toenails clean. The natural color of nails can indicate how your system is coping during and after surgery. It makes no sense to camouflage them with makeup.

The night before my wife's surgery, someone, maybe it was the anaesthetist, came in to talk with her. He delivered a descriptive monologue, followed by a question-and-answer session, on the next morning's procedure. It was meant to help put both our minds at ease. His parting remark did just the opposite.

It was 1984. Everyone charged with collecting and distributing blood, from government health people to the Canadian Red Cross Society, was saying there was zero danger of contracting AIDS from transfusions.

Not so, we were told, almost as an afterthought. As if my

wife's facing major surgery the next morning weren't stress enough, we were advised that she ran the risk of being infected with HIV-tainted blood.

The shock must have shown on our faces.

"It's a very small risk," the doctor said quickly. "Don't worry about it. I have to mention it . . . " he lamely added " . . . to absolve the hospital of legal responsibility."

Today, eleven years later, despite the shameful coverup by government and health agencies, ongoing hearings and settlements reveal how very real and present that risk was and to some extent still is.

My wife went into surgery early the next morning. I was waiting in her room with her when they came in with the gurney.

"Ready?" asked the nurse in charge.

I felt Chris was wondering what would happen if she were totally honest and said no. Not now. Not ever.

Instead, she put on a smiling show of bravado and nodded. With just a little help, she rolled herself onto the gurney. I recognized it as the kind of small statement she typically would make. She was saying that she could still do some things for herself.

I took her hand in mine and gave her a kiss. "I'll be waiting for you right here," I said. "Hurry back."

It was not until that evening that Chris was returned to her room from the post-op or recovery room, and I was allowed a brief visit. She told me later that her body felt like it was stuffed with sharp shards of glass and cotton batting. She said where she didn't hurt she couldn't feel. It took her some time to get her mouth working so she could speak. Her first efforts didn't make sense. The one word she finally managed was less than a whisper.

With her hand in mine, I brought my ear close to her lips to hear.

"Col . . . os . . . tomy?"

A nurse was adjusting the intravenous. I glanced at her and phrased the word soundlessly. She smiled and shook her head.

"No," I said. "You don't have a colostomy."

Chris said something I couldn't make out, but relief showed in her eyes. She told me later that what she had tried to say was "Thank God! Thank God for small mercies!"

She dropped off to sleep soon after, and I left. What I figured my wife needed right then, and the nurse agreed, was all the R and R—rest and recovery—that she could get.

I arrived the next morning with a bouquet of brave spring flowers, adding to the growing floral display by her bed. She was still very much in recovery, but more with it than she had been the previous day. She remembered my visit. She also told me of the odd last thought she had had before she had fallen asleep.

"I thought of how my body had been scarred by the operation," she said.

She hadn't been upset by this. It had just, in some strange way, made her a little sad.

While we were talking, Arnold Rogers showed up on his morning rounds. Before we saw him, we heard his deep voice and laughter as he paused to joke with someone in the corridor outside my wife's room. He breezed in, followed by a nurse with a clipboard.

"How are you this morning?"

My wife grimaced. "I'm having a lot of pain."

Dr. Rogers glanced inquiringly at the nurse with the poised clipboard.

She nodded. "She is. The medication's not holding her."

The grin Dr. Rogers had brought into the room disappeared. He was suddenly, surprisingly angry. "Damnit!" he bellowed. "Tell him to give her more."

The nurse almost dropped her pencil. She nodded again and quickly jotted down something on her clipboard. "Him" apparently was whoever had prescribed the amount of pain-killer Chris was to be given.

There is a big advantage to having a doctor who knows about pain. Many of them don't. Many have never experienced and have no understanding of the degree of pain their patients experience, and have never bothered to learn about it. Dr. Rogers had first-hand knowledge. As a boy, he had suffered from a chronic intestinal illness. He was bed-ridden for more than a year and has undergone a dozen or so major surgeries. One of these was a colostomy.

The problem of pain relief out of the way, he was clearly pleased with himself. He sat on the edge of the bed and took my wife's hand. "You're lucky I'm suspicious by nature," he said. "You can thank me for insisting on that second set of tests."

Dr. Broder had done a frozen-section biopsy at the beginning of Chris' surgery. The results, rushed to the hospital lab while she was still on the table, had confirmed Dr. Rogers' suspicions. Her tumor was malignant.

The pain got worse the second day.

"And I thought giving birth was tough!" Chris gasped between spasms. She likened having each of our three sons to "child's play" (this with a tight grin) compared to the gas pains she was suffering from her colon resection.

Dr. Broder had removed part of the colon, which is the large intestine, with the tumor. If it had been benign, he simply would have cut the tumor out at its base. Because it was malignant, he had also taken surrounding tissue in case that, too, had diseased cells. Then he had stitched together her shortened colon.

I sat in a chair by the bed so I wouldn't give Chris any more discomfort than she already had. I cast around for something positive to say.

"Broder thinks he got it all."

"When did he say that?"

"Right after your surgery. When you were still in the recovery room."

"Did he tell you anything else?"

"He said a malignant tumor is like a stone bedded in pebbles. When you dig out the stone, you hope to get all the pebbles, too. He thinks he did."

I thought back to my talk with Morris Broder. "He also told me you were lucky. The tumor hadn't penetrated the wall."

"What wall?"

During my wife's surgery, I had been waiting in a small lounge off the corridor that led from the operating room. Dr. Broder and I had spoken just moments after members of his support team had charged past me with Chris lying deathly pale and terribly still on the gurney. Any questions I normally might have asked were awash in a flood of relief that my wife had survived the operation.

Now I looked at her blankly. "He didn't say. I assume he meant the intestinal wall."

Chris told me on my next visit that while I had gone on speaking, she hadn't been hearing me. She was in a state of shock. "My God," she said, "neither of us was even sure what Broder was talking about!"

She blamed herself.

She said she realized none of her doctors had the time, even if they wanted to, to discuss her disease with her, and the procedures involved, as fully as she wished. Even if one did, she felt that she would be getting only one opinion, one person's expertise, on an illness and its treatment that was highly complex and controversial.

She also began having disturbing thoughts. She had read somewhere that the seeds of cancer are in everyone. She questioned why hers had taken root. She wondered if she could have been at least partly responsible.

A few days after she came home from the hospital, Chris announced that she had a need to know. "Not just exactly what my tumor didn't penetrate," she said, "but everything else I can find out about this damned disease!"

I was just as determined to be my wife's active partner. Not only in her quest for answers, but in providing whatever it took to help her cope with living with cancer.

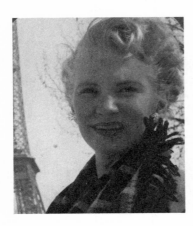

Return to Paris. Summer '58 — *Escalope de veau* had been a favorite entrée at a family café called *La Bonne Table* when we were first married and living in Paris. There had been few problems then. Certainly none like the one we faced now.

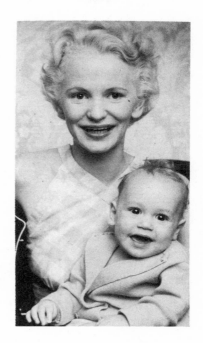

With second son, Casey. Summer '55 — She had been a healthy, privileged and generally happy person all her life. How and why, she had wondered aloud, can this be happening?

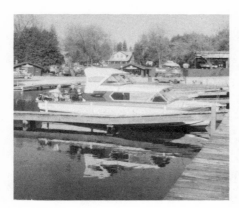

The yacht. Summer '63 — The breached hull began taking on buckets of water. In the confusion, I heard my wife call out to the kids: "Strip the bunks and fold your bedding!" That's the way she was. If we were going to sink, by golly, we were going to sink neat!

2·Learning about the enemy

Would she ever feel whole again?

Chris doubted it.

Her very determined day nurse made her work at it. A couple of days after my wife's surgery, while I helped a little apprehensively, she coaxed Chris out of bed and we eased her into a chair. The next morning I found the nurse and a student, one on each arm, helping her shuffle down the corridor. The following day, looking quite proud of herself, Chris met me at the elevator near the nursing station.

She was walking slowly, pulling along the wheeled tripod with dangling "IV" bottle which steadily drips intravenous fluid down a thin plastic hose to a vein in the arm.

"Meet my boyfriend," she said.

They got along pretty well together, which was good, since the "boyfriend" had to go everywhere she did. Within a few days they made it down to the hospital hair salon for what Chris had decided was a desperately needed wash and set.

I had to agree that the hairdo she had gotten just before entering hospital was a wreck. Post-operative sweats and days and nights of head-tossing on pillows will do that. She said she thought shampoo and a blow-dry might give the Inner Woman a lift.

"As well as those who have to look at the Outer Woman," she added.

Unlike some hospitals, The Misery at that time was not big on treating the outer look of the Inner Woman. Its hair salon did not have blow-driers. Soon after, in what I assume male board members saw as a further cutback on the vanities, it eliminated the shop altogether.

Chris's hair was set in rollers and she was seated under a floor-drier.

In just a few minutes, she realized this was a mistake. In recalling why, she told me she abruptly realized she could not sit still, for one second longer, under this thing.

"I was in sheer panic," she said.

She ducked out from under the drier, took hold of her "boyfriend," and together they trundled over to the surprised hairdresser.

"I can't wait!" Chris blurted out. She figured the woman could take this any way she wanted.

She took it as an emergency. In moments she had whipped the rollers out of my wife's wet hair and was steering her towards the door.

Chris and I later shared a laugh over this. "Whatever 'can't wait' kind of emergency it was," Chris said, "it sure wasn't going to happen in her salon!"

What had created the situation itself wasn't laughable.

"The worst part wasn't that I felt and knew I looked like a drowned rat. Or that my legs were shaky all the way back to my room. It was the realization that I had panicked for no apparent reason in a perfectly normal situation.

"It came home to me with a shock that somewhere along the way my psyche had slipped a key."

As she climbed back into bed, she knew that she had an emotional recovery to make that was at least equal to the physical one.

"It was a scary end," she said, "to something as simple as a botched hairdo."

When Chris, on the drive to The Misery, had asked for the umpteenth time if her doctors had told me anything they hadn't told her, we had experienced the paranoia cancer breeds. We were now seeing that it also could create unpredictable, unreasoning flashes of panic.

Chris was discharged eleven days after her surgery. I came for her just before noon. Her day nurse took her down to the hospital entrance and out to the curb in a wheelchair. I had packed her few things in the "happy bag" and put it in the trunk. She had asked me to keep the "Get well" cards, so she could acknowledge them, but to leave behind her collection of florists' flower vases, wicker fruit baskets, and a long-lasting bouquet.

Chris had decided she did not want these mementos of her stay at The Misery. She wanted those last eleven days of her life to be history.

As I helped her up from the wheelchair, her day nurse impulsively leaned forward and kissed her on the forehead. "Good luck," she said.

Chris thanked her, but when we pulled away from the curb she made a wry face. "Does she think I'll need it?"

Just that morning we had discussed the cancer patient's proclivity to think those around them, out of mistaken kindness, are holding back on their actual condition. She had made me promise, now and always, to be honest with her. I gave her what I hoped was a reassuring grin. "Your paranoia is showing."

"I hope that's all it is."

She said that nothing inside her felt right. Everything still hurt. She had been told that her body would be back to normal in six weeks. She had already worked that out on a mental calendar. As soon as we got home, she planned to circle May 20 on the one that hung by her kitchen desk.

We drove back over the Maryland Bridge and took the scenic route along Wellington Crescent. It seemed like almost forever since we had played hooky from checking into The Misery and lunched at the Courtyard Café.

After its Siberian winter, Winnipeg is a city of many heaved streets and potholes. I drove slowly, managing to miss most of them. After a particularly bad jolt, we both grimaced; I in sympathy. "Okay?" I asked. Chris nodded. I could tell from her tight-lipped look that she was hurting too much to reply.

The potholes weren't her only problem. She was wearing the skirt with elasticized waistband, trying to keep it from squeezing her lower abdomen.

"Drive faster," she said. "I've got to get out of this damned skirt!"

She was half out of it by the time she limped through the house and got to the bedroom closet. Looking for anything that was loose-fitting, she chose a black wool dress that she could wear without the belt.

I brought her a walking-stick from the front hall. Fashioned from stout mountain ash and knobbed at the handle, it is a souvenir of a year we spent living in the Laurentians, near St-Sauveur.

The thought of carrying what I call my "Quebec shille-lagh" made Chris laugh.

"I'm serious. You may need this for a while."

She took a determined few steps to show me how wrong I was. She already had been too long on her feet for her first day out of hospital. She lurched sideways. I grabbed her arm to keep her from falling.

I must have had one of those "I-told-you-so" looks on my face, because I sensed that Chris wanted to slug me with my Quebec shillelagh. Instead, she took it and steadied herself.

"Okay," she said. "but just until I get my sealegs back."

She stumped out to the kitchen and took a marker pen from her desk drawer. Then she raised the April sheet and circled and made an entry under May 20.

"Six weeks," she wrote. "All better!"

We had decided in hospital to find out all we could about colon cancer. Until Chris was able to get out and go to the library, our only source was one of those do-it-yourself medi-cal books that we had been sent with a subscription to some-thing or other. It's the sort of thing, up-dated, that well-meaning missionaries used to take with them to places like Darkest Africa.

Together we looked up colon cancer. It was given eight-een lines under "Signs and Symptoms," some of which we now recognized all too well. Unfortunately, they could sug-gest equally anything from food poisoning and Hong Kong flu to hemorrhoids.

What shook us both up was the chapter heading.

"The Killers."

In Chris's state of mind, that was all she needed. She was paranoid enough as it was.

A number of close friends and relatives came to visit Chris

her first week back home. The first were her brother, Don, and his wife, Pam.

Winnipeg was inching into spring and the weather was growing sunny and warmer.

"I want to look sprightly, too," Chris said. "Not grey and gaunt like someone who's just had cancer surgery is supposed to look!"

She chose to wear a black-and-white print crepe dress, loose-fitting. She still couldn't tolerate anything that put any pressure on her waist. She knew that, all things considered, she looked pretty good. She had lost weight, but not too much. "A few pounds," Chris said, "that I could well afford to lose."

Oddly enough, her green eyes seemed somehow larger, but this was a definite plus.

Standing in front of her dressmaker's mirror, she liked the overall effect. It obviously gave her a lift. The pain from her surgery, still always present, seemed a little diminished. She had a hostess role to play. She was determined to play it well.

Pam and Chris had had their differences. No more nor less than most in-laws, I imagine, or siblings for that matter, but they always basically had been good friends. One thing I don't recall their ever being was demonstrative towards each other.

I opened the door to Don and Pam. They came in looking a little awkward, something Chris noticed, too.

A few months down the road, Chris and I both came to realize how tough it is for most people to relate casually to someone with cancer.

"It's almost like visiting someone on death row." she said. "Appeals may keep you alive a while. A full pardon, though always possible, is unlikely. It's hard for them to know how to act and what to say."

I had to agree with her. It's not that easy to be casual when you feel you're looking someone else's death in the face. Especially when that face belongs to someone close to you.

Chris hadn't yet learned this from her own experience, so it threw her when Pam abruptly stepped forward, embraced her, and kissed her on the cheek.

My wife's surprise gave way to yet another flash of paranoia. She gave me a quick, almost accusing look. I could read what she was thinking. *What does she know that I don't? Do I have just a few weeks to live? A few days maybe—and everybody knows but me?*

Her brother Don was speaking.

"You look just great," he said. He turned to his wife. "Doesn't she look just great, Pam?"

"She certainly does," said Pam.

Chris said after they'd left that she loved them for their underlying concern. She also didn't believe a word they said. For a while, she didn't believe me, either. She was convinced that her family, friends, and doctors were all part of a conspiracy, and that I was right at the heart of it.

More than anything else, Chris wanted to get to a library, where she could research her condition. She felt that only from this impersonal source could she get the facts that would also bring her peace of mind.

Another frustrating week went by. She still was not well enough to leave the house. She was taking a lot of Tylenol 3, which had been prescribed "as needed" for pain. The only way she could sit comfortably was perched on the edge of a chair.

Our three cats—Fraidy, Mad Maggie, and S'Puss S'Puss— were used to jumping up onto my wife's lap. You can imagine the sudden and unexpected shock. Each was sent scurrying, stopping only to look back reproachfully, after being yelled at and dumped on the floor.

Chris moved about the house gingerly, helped along by my Quebec shillelagh. She was counting the days to May 20, when she would be "all better."

She hadn't had her hair done since before her surgery. She said that the disaster at the hairdresser's at The Misery didn't count. Ten days after she got home, she felt well enough to pay a visit to Mario at his salon in Polo Park Mall. Again he rose to the occasion and worked her in on just overnight notice.

A few years earlier, I had been doing some European corresponding for newspapers. We had spent a month or so in Rome and on the Island of Capri as guests of the famed Italian actress, Gina Lollobrigida, and her sister-in-law, Dada Skofic. Ever since, my wife had had a soft spot in her heart for Italian men.

"They're not just romantics," she said, after setting up her next morning's appointment with Mario. "Italian men have a practical side that recognizes when a woman needs all the help she can get!"

I parked the car as close as I could to the mall's main entrance. Mario's salon is just the second location inside the doors. Before we got there, Chris was walking with some difficulty, even with my Quebec shillelagh. I took her by the arm.

"Are you going to be okay?"

She nodded, keeping her eyes on the floor. Knowing her as well as I did, I knew what she was thinking.

How I hate limping along like this, poking my stick ahead of me and leaning on my husband like some damned invalid!

When she decided she wanted to talk about it, Chris told me how she saw herself. She said it was as though she were standing off to one side, watching this person who was someone else. This wasn't the world-class shopper who loped through Polo Park once a week, checking for new arrivals at Holt Renfrew and Eaton's and all the little boutiques on two levels. This wasn't the real her. Her strong, supple body had been put into a check-room when she'd entered the operating room at The Misery. This old, broken-down replacement had been given her by mistake.

"Hi, Mrs. Edge . . . I'll be with you in a minute!"

Chris unhooked herself from my arm and returned Mario's bright smile.

Apparently it wasn't obvious to anyone but her that she was walking around in the wrong body.

An hour-and-a-half later, we met in the public sitting area adjacent to Mario's. I had been browsing around the mall.

"Your hair looks great!" I said.

Chris knew I meant it. Mario always did a terrific job. Finally getting her hair done and my obvious pleasure with how she looked gave her a lift.

"Let's do the shops," she said.

I didn't think she was yet up to it. "You're sure?"

"We'll walk to the Eaton's entrance and come back on the second level."

Eaton's is at the other end of the mall.

I hesitated.

"We can go slow," Chris urged.

There are benches at regular intervals along the main floor to Eaton's. We stopped at all of them. When we reached the entrance to the department store, Chris knew that she'd had enough. "I don't think I can make it back."

I helped her to a nearby bench. "I'll go and bring the car around."

I knew she was embarrassed with herself.

"I'm sorry," she said.

"What's to be sorry for?" I squeezed her hand before turning to go for the car. "I'll just be a few minutes."

Ever since leaving the hospital, Chris had been growing more frustrated and angrier with her cancer and what it was doing to her.

"Anger with your disease is good," Dr. McIntyre had told her, during a visit to the house just that week. "But only if it's directed without, not within."

On the drive home, Chris told me that while she was waiting for me to bring the car around, she had been thinking about what Don McIntyre had said.

"Feeling miserable in Polo Park Mall is a long way from getting a good, positive mad on. If I'm going to be honest with myself, it may be more like self-pity."

"I think you're being a little hard on yourself," I said.

"Maybe. But feeling sorry for myself won't get me anywhere but down."

Recovering from surgery in The Misery, Chris had promised herself to find out everything she could about her disease. This had been put on hold by the business of getting home and trying to get back on her feet again. She decided that it was now time to keep that promise.

"With all the support I've been getting from you and Don McIntyre," she said, "I'm still the person most responsible for me. When are you going back to the library?"

For some months, I had been doing what seemed like never-ending research on the biography of Dr. Charlotte Ross. I had been mining information daily, in Winnipeg's Centennial Library, from the microfilmed pages of newspapers published in Winnipeg in the 1800's. I had done little work on the book since Chris had undergone surgery.

"I don't know," I said. "When you're feeling better."

"Tomorrow," Chris said, "I'll go with you. I really have to start getting out more often."

"You're sure you won't be overdoing it?"

I caught the look Chris gave me. She didn't say anything, but more than once over the past while I had caught that small frown of annoyance.

I was the kind of husband who makes spontaneous little statements to his wife: a kiss on the back of the neck, a light squeeze of an arm or a hand, an unexpected embrace. Chris used to tease me that I romanticized an Italian ancestor in some ancient branch of my English-Irish family tree.

From the day we learned she had cancer, I had been making these gestures more often. I had meant them to be reassuring. I was not aware that their effect on Chris had been just the opposite. They were telling her that I was just as frightened and confused as she was.

On top of that, I had protested the unsuccessful walk in the mall. Now I was questioning whether she was well enough to go with me to the library. A few days earlier, I had come home to find her tentatively vacuuming the living-room carpet. I had quickly crossed the floor and tried to take over. "Here," I protested, "let me do that."

Almost angrily, she pushed me away.

"For God's sake," she said, "I can still do my own vacuuming!"

The learning process had begun for me too. It came with the realization that lending too much love and support can be almost as bad as offering none at all. How could she find out what her limits were without testing them?

"Okay," I agreed. "The library tomorrow morning."

Over the next couple of months, Chris spent almost as

much time at the Winnipeg Centennial Library as I did. We arrived just as it opened at 10:00 a.m., leaving the car in its underground parking and taking the elevator so Chris wouldn't have far to walk.

She was still using my Quebec shillelagh. Adhesions are the painful aftermath of the internal surgery she had undergone. They occur when the inflamed walls of organs adhere to each other. She concluded that this common post-operative problem caused her as much grief, over her lengthy convalescence, as the surgery itself.

I had resumed researching my biography of Dr. Charlotte Ross. I spent my days on the library's mezzanine in front of a microfilm machine. I was getting square eyes from reading and jotting down bits and pieces of information from newspapers from the 1800s-on, projected onto a monitor.

Below, on the main floor, Chris sat at a table surrounded by books on cancer—reading, digesting, and making rafts of notes. She was a skilled researcher. After attending United College, now part of the University of Winnipeg, she had become a journalist. With her family grown, she had made a new career for herself as an award-winning fashion writer, TV advertising writer-producer, and Director of Special Promotions for Eaton's West.

At noon, we met in the library's cafeteria-style lunchroom and discussed her morning's notes over a Saran-wrapped salad and a tea. The room was smoke-free, which was fine with us. Both heavy smokers for many years, we had stopped when we realized we were paying dearly at both ends—the high cost of cigarettes and the certainty that we were setting ourselves up for lung and heart disease.

As young people, our lifestyle role models had been people like Bogart, Bergman, and Bacall, in movies like *Casa-*

blanca and Ernest Hemingway's *To Have and Have Not.* In such popular flicks, the macho hero and sexy heroine always had a glass in one hand and a cigarette in the other.

In the same time-frame, saturation advertising told us that the "Man of Distinction" drank Seagram's whiskey and to "Be happy, go Lucky" by smoking Lucky Strike cigarettes.

Chris's favorite cookbook was Roy Andries de Groot's *Feasts for All Seasons*, possibly American cuisine's greatest compilation of gourmet recipes, calories, and cholesterol.

It doesn't appear to be that much different now. American TV commercials tell us that the sexiest young people having the most fun drink a lot of chemically brewed beer. While they may be killing themselves in the process, too many teenagers, apparently girls in particular, are picking up on the cigarette habit. And you can stuff yourself with calories and cholesterol, without bothering with an Andries de Groot gourmet dinner, at any one of the hundreds of fast food outlets.

Since Chris had begun reading up on cancer, she had cut out the Scotches we had shared—had given up pretty well all alcohol, in fact, except for the occasional sherry, or glass of white wine with dinner, which she enjoyed. I also had seen a subtle change in what she ordered when we ate out and what she put on the table at home: more broiled and boiled foods instead of fried. Smaller portions of meat, with more fish dishes. More salads. Simple fruit desserts instead of outrageously rich ones—like her famous amaretto cheesecake, which all our friends said was "to die for!"

To which my wife now added: "Not literally, I hope."

At our luncheon at the Courtyard Café, before checking into The Misery, Chris had wondered aloud: "How can this be happening? Other people get cancer. Other people die from it. Not me."

"I'm finding out that an awful lot of 'other people' get cancer," she said. "One in three Canadians."

She made a face. "Of which I am now one."

She described cancer, in simple terms, as a disease caused by renegade cells that grow abnormally, displacing and destroying normal ones.

"As for causes," Chris said, "some are known, most are just guessed at. For everything I'm finding out there that's black and white, there's an awful lot of grey!"

She gave me a few "for instances."

"It's accepted by just about everybody but the tobacco companies that smoking can cause lung cancer. Some oncologists believe that alcohol abuse can lead to cancer. It's generally agreed that a diet heavy in fats and rich foods can. Farm crops treated with some pesticides are suspect, as are some food additives. Emotional stress may be a factor, and some cancers, like colon, may run in the family."

Chris looked her confusion. "At the same time, non-smokers, non-drinkers, vegetarians and children get cancer. Some infants, too. Apparently the seeds of cancer are in all of us.

"Why do they take root in some and not others? No one really knows."

She read from another page of her notes. She prefaced it with the remark that because it's so difficult to determine and correlate cancer statistics, they almost always come qualified by the word "estimated."

Estimated or not, the figures shocked me, as they did her.

"It's estimated that more than a half-million people in Canada have cancer," Chris read. "There are more than one hundred thousand new cases annually, and that figure's steadily rising."

She explained that one of the reasons for this is that the older you get, the more chance you have of getting some form of cancer. Since more people are living longer, there has been a corresponding increase in cases.

"There also has been a corresponding increase in deaths," she said. "An estimated fifty to sixty thousand each year."

Taking breast cancer as one specific example, she said that one in nine women will get breast cancer. One in twenty-three will die from it.

"Breast and lung cancer are the two leading causes of women's deaths from cancer. Colon,"—Chris read off another fact—"is third, followed by ovarian."

For men, prostate cancer, named for the generative organ gland, is said to be the major killer, followed by lung and colon.

"For both men and women," Chris added, "the chances of getting cancer and dying from it are much higher at fifty years and beyond.

May 20 came and went and Chris still wasn't "all better." Far from it.

The adhesions from her surgery were giving her hell. The battery of doctors she was now seeing weren't sure what the problem was.

Beginning in mid-April, they had put Chris on what she called "a not-so-merry-go-round" of tests, X-ray, and medications. Her primary physician, Dr. McIntyre, thought that the severe stomach pain she was suffering might be from an ulcer.

"After all you've been through," he told her, "it wouldn't surprise me."

He sent Chris to see her surgeon, Morris Broder, who prescribed the ulcer drug Tagamet.

One morning soon after, I got up before Chris and whipped together some fluffy scrambled eggs with chopped chives, a favorite of hers. I called out to her that breakfast was ready. She didn't answer.

I found her perched on the edge of the bed, looking scared. "I can't walk," she said.

Dr. McIntyre arrived, and together, back and forth across the living-room, we helped her walk off whatever it was that had immobilized her. McIntyre prescribed Prednisone, an anti-inflammatory drug, which he thought might help. She didn't have any more trouble walking, but she began to have side effects: chronic stomach and intestinal upset, combined with dizziness and frequent periods of seeing "black spots."

On one of our days at the library, she discovered that Prednisone is also a chemotherapy drug. She mentioned this to me almost casually in the lunchroom.

"I'm not thrilled to find that out," she said, "but it hasn't panicked me the way it would have a few months ago. Like most people, I think that as long as I know, I can cope."

I had always admired my wife's determination to make the best of what was, a determination she once attributed to "my stolid Scottish roots!" That respect had grown since we had first learned she had cancer. It would continue to do so over the rough times ahead.

Since nothing seemed to be getting much better, she wondered if the original cancer had begun to metastasize, the oncology word for spread. McIntyre said he didn't think so, but suggested that he set up an appointment for her with Arnold Rogers.

Chris had begun to realize the importance of making

notes on her current condition and listing what questions she wanted answered by her doctors.

Rogers had told her early in their relationship, "I'll answer any questions you have." To which Chris had replied, "Yes, but I have to know the questions to ask, don't I?"

She found it difficult but important to describe accurately where she felt pain and what type it was: Dull? Sharp? Short? Long-lasting? Chest? Stomach? Left side? Right?

Chris and Rogers got along well together. This was their first meeting since she had begun researching cancer and making lists.

When she began describing in detail the pain she was suffering, leading to the questions she had listed, Rogers pushed back in his chair. "You're starting to sound like a Jewish princess!" he boomed.

Chris took that as a compliment. She figured that it marked the end of her role as a passive patient. She had begun to put herself front and centre when it came to her own medical health care.

Over June and July, and then again through September, Chris had an ongoing series of diagnostic appointments with Rogers, McIntyre, and a specialist in gynecology in the Medical Arts building. They all knew something was wrong. None was sure what. Adhesions? Ulcer? Metastasis? Kidney stone? She was given blood tests, liver tests, and bone scans. The appointment with the gynecologist was set up to check for the possibility of a simple yeast infection, or perhaps some more serious gynecological problem.

In between, Chris continued her visits to the library.

"What I'm getting," she said, "is that cancer is a very complex disease. In fact, some oncologists think that it may be many different complex diseases."

She named some of them for me: Cancer of the breast. Leukemia (of the blood). Melanoma (of the skin). Lymphoma (of the lymph nodes, a vital part of the body's disease defence system). Larynx (of the throat). Cervix and Uterus (of the female reproductive organs). Brain. Bladder. Stomach. Kidney. Liver.

"Those are some of the more commonly known ones," she said.

It surprised me, as it had her, that there are more than one hundred different types of cancer.

"Doctors use a 'stage' system," Chris read from her notes, "to measure the severity of the disease.

"It's a little more involved than this, but in general terms Stage I describes an early tumor that hasn't yet metastasized. In Stage II, it has spread to underlying tissue, but not beyond. It has reached Stage III when the cancer cells have invaded adjacent organs or lymph nodes. Stage IV is the final stage, when malignant cells have spread to random parts of the body and the patient has advanced cancer.

"For colon cancer, the stages range from O to IV, with A's and B's," Chris said. "And to complicate things further, there's also a Dukes' system of staging, escalating from Dukes' A to Dukes' D."

We had been told that my wife's cancer had been Stage IA, or Dukes' A. This meant that if Broder had "gotten it all," as he said he thought he had, it had not yet spread to underlying tissue.

All we could do now was wait and see.

Chris and I had a lot of discussions about this, and about the controversial and often conflicting paths along which her research was taking her.

"All those 'estimated' statistics and percentages on cancer can lead you every-which-way," she said at one point. "It often depends on who's presenting them and for what reason."

Shortly after her surgery, Broder had told Chris that the percentage chance she had of being free of cancer was "60-40," to which she had replied, "Well, I guess that's better than the other way around." She knew now that this was just a figure that Broder had pulled out of his caring physician's hope chest.

"You can't fault someone for wanting to give a cancer patient hope," she said. "When you lose that, you've lost everything. I just wish more people understood that giving false hope can be just as devastating as giving none at all."

The more Chris learned about cancer, the more she spoke openly about it.

"I refuse to treat it like some dirty little secret," she said. "I haven't got some unspeakable social disease."

She told me that after her surgery, even her nurse at The Misery had avoided the use of the word "cancer." When Chris talked about it among our family and friends, I couldn't help but notice that it made them feel uncomfortable.

We liked to give elaborate little dinner parties, Saturday evenings in our own home, for four. Chris would spend the afternoon fussing over the table settings and centrepiece, usually one that reflected the season. Then, having made dessert the night before, she would do the appetizers. The main course was my responsibility. I enjoyed banging frypans and pots around, perhaps juggling a flaming entrée with a couple or three vegetables, artfully (I hoped!) making it all come together at the same time.

After dinner, we sat in the living-room and talked.

At one of these dinner parties, Chris began talking about

information on cancer that she had just dug up at the library. Her friend's husband, obviously unable to bring himself to use the word cancer in front of Chris, said something about "the Big 'C.'"

"For God's sake," she exploded, "say it! Cancer! C-A-N-C-E-R!"

I understood what she was doing. If she had to live with this disease, she had to talk about it. Openly. Not to the point of boring everyone to tears, literally, but enough to acknowledge that she had cancer and was doing her best to cope with it. It was a kind of therapy.

A big part of that, in the long run, was her refusal to be considered a "victim."

"People almost always refer to cancer patients as 'victims,'" she protested. "Why? No one talks about 'heart victims,' or 'diabetes victims,' or 'pneumonia victims.'"

Without realizing it, I had been guilty of that myself. I had not been aware, until then, how much Chris hated this term that defined cancer patients as helplessly at the mercy of their disease.

Both my wife and I became conscious of the barbs, in everyday news reports, that make some people with cancer uncomfortable: "Drug trafficking is a cancer in our society." "Graft and corruption are cancers in our political system." "It is evil, like a cancer." "It must be cut out like a cancer."

Chris had a quip for this kind of thing. "Cancer isn't just a killer," she said. "It's an embarrassment."

Cancer patients often find humor in their condition in conversations with those closest to them and with other cancer patients. It's a kind of black humor. It falls flat with people who don't have cancer or are not that close to someone who does.

Eventually, Chris and I got involved with someone who had written a book some years earlier about his own experience with cancer. He titled it for the way a friend he hadn't seen for some time had greeted him at a chance meeting in downtown Vancouver: "My God!" his friend had cried out. "I thought you'd died!"

The book was sent to Chris by Marion Hensley, a friend from her schoolgirl days who had married and moved to Edmonton. She and Chris had kept in touch over the years. Marion sent the book when she learned that Chris had cancer. The title is a come-on. It actually is a very positive book. Marion thought that it might help her old friend a little. In a more personal way than she could have imagined, it did.

By early fall, six months after her surgery, Chris was having better days and more of them. She wasn't in as much chronic pain as she'd been, and she had happily ditched my Quebec shillelagh.

The Banff Centre is an arts complex, itself state-of-the-art, just outside the town of Banff, in the Rockies. It provides accommodations, recreational facilities, and instruction in music, theatre, and the visual, media, and literary arts. Serious students enrol from all over the world.

Part of the complex is the Leighton Artist Colony, where I had been a resident writer the previous year. A scattering of six comfortable and functional cabins are set off by themselves in the woods. They are available to established artists, musicians, and writers with a work in progress that the Colony board endorses.

It had been the perfect place for me to work on my book, which I had just begun writing. I decided we should return to Banff for a visit. After such a tough year, I thought it would be good for Chris just to sit back and relax in the glorious fall setting of the Canadian Rockies.

There was a small hitch at the last moment. We had hired a young woman to sit the house, our two black Standard Poodles, Beau and Ms. Liz, and Fraidy, S'Puss S'Puss, and Mad Maggie. When she came to take over, I saw that she had misgivings.

After much humming and hawing, I finally got it out of her that she was afraid of catching my wife's "disease." She carefully avoided the use of the word "cancer." With our cab due at any moment, I did a hard-sell job that cancer is not contagious. There never has been any evidence that contact with a cancer patient, no matter how intimate (let alone just the house in which she lives!) can give someone cancer.

The next couple of weeks were everything I'd hoped they'd be. Chris was able to relax fully for the first time since her surgery. She didn't have any pain, or if she did she didn't speak of it, and we took frequent walks together around Banff and the Centre itself. As well as a gym and a pool, its recreational facility offers the warmth and hospitality of a common room bar with a large island fireplace. There is a weekly menu of music concerts and movie nights.

Best of all, we were both caught up in the youthful optimism, ambition, and dedication to their art—the pure love of life—of the young people at the Centre. It was just what Chris needed.

She was well-rested and in good spirits when we returned to Winnipeg.

Chris had a prearranged appointment with Arnold Rogers at his office in the Doctors Building.

After a brief question-and-answer period that covered everything from Banff to aches-and-pains, Rogers prepared to usher us out. "Now don't hold me to this," he said to Chris, "but I think you could be a cure."

It took a moment for my wife to react to this.

"You do?"

"Well, just look at you. Your eyes are sparkling and you look really well!"

When we reached the street, Chris gave me a broad smile. "You know," she said, "for the first time, I really do feel all better."

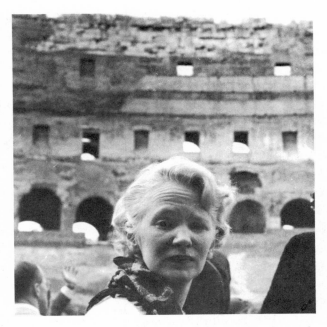

The Coliseum, Summer '58 — We had spent a month or so in Rome and on the Island of Capri as guests of the famed Italian actress Gina Lollobrigida and her sister-in-law, Dada Skofic. Ever since, my wife had had a soft spot in her heart for Italian men.

Chris in her teens.
Winnipeg '41 — As young people, our lifestyle role models had been people like Bogart, Bergman, and Bacall, in movies like *Casablanca* and Ernest Hemingway's *To Have and Have Not.* The macho hero and sexy heroine always had a glass in one hand and a cigarette in the other.

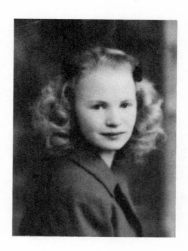

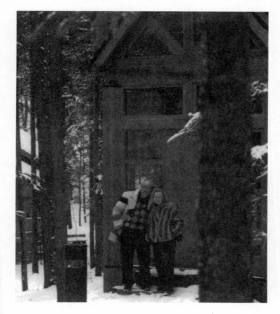

The Leighton Artist Colony, Banff Centre.
Fall '84 — We were both caught up in the youthful optimism, ambition, and dedication to their art— the pure love of life—of the young people at the Centre. It was just what Chris needed.

3 · "All better!"

Although she felt a lot more like her old self, Chris continued to read everything about cancer she could get her hands on.

She soon discovered that it's common practice for doctors to put a spin on plain English when they're discussing the disease with their patients.

"It's probably well-intentioned," she said, "but that doesn't make it any less deceitful. For those of us who don't want to live in a fool's paradise, there should be a special 'book of phrases' for cancer patients."

She translated a few of the more common ones for me.

"All better" was the state she was in now, some eight months, not six weeks, after her discharge from The Misery; able, for all practical purposes, to resume the life she had led before surgery.

"I knew so little then that I took what I was told at face value. I actually thought that 'all better' meant that I was going to be just that—feeling great and free of cancer."

Arnold Rogers had said that, while he didn't want Chris to hold him to it, he thought she "could be a cure."

"'Cured' is the term with the greatest spin on it," she said. "It's used to express five-year survival rates. What it actually means is that the patient probably has been 'cured' for five years. If their cancer hasn't recurred by the end of that time, their 'cure' might last another five years. And so on."

"That's when it's said to be in remission," I offered, since I'd heard the term before.

"Maybe. Maybe not," Chris replied. "It may be in actual remission. This means that there's no longer any evidence of cancer, though dormant cancer cells may still be in the body.

"Partial remission is when the cancer appears to be inactive, but there are still some symptoms.

"Or, it may not be in remission at all. An indolent cancer is a slow-growing one that may cause little discomfort and show few symptoms.

"What we cancer patients have to be realistic about," said Chris, "is that anyone can have a recurrence after their surgery, whether or not it's followed by chemotherapy or radiation. It may be soon after. It may be some years later."

This brought us full circle to my wife's surgery and Morris Broder's comment that he thought he had "got it all." Chris now understood that he had cut out the main mass of the tumor in her colon, and, she hoped, enough diseased surrounding tissue to delay a recurrence.

"None of my doctors was lying to me," she said. "They were just not telling me the truth by speaking a language I didn't understand. I suppose it's seen as a way of holding out hope. I'd rather have known the truth and handled the hope part myself."

The truth is that so far we have lost the war on cancer, officially declared almost fifty years ago by the late President Richard Nixon. Despite massive funding for research and treatment in the United States, proportionately matched in Canada and many other countries, no one yet has conquered this disease that pre-dates the pyramids. For the most part, cancer appears to be almost as invincible an enemy today as it was to the ancient Egyptians.

The only bright side has been the death rate among children. This has dropped dramatically over the past twenty years or so, despite an increase in incidence. Largely responsible have been earlier diagnosis and improved treatment of children's leukemia and lymphoma.

The death rate for adults continues to rise. This is despite the fact that the National Cancer Institute in the United States spends more than one-and-a-half billion dollars each year on research. Canada spends more than $70 million.

John Bailar is a member of McGill University's medical faculty, in Montreal, and scholar-in-residence at the United States National Academy of Science. Writing on cancer in the journal *Chronic Diseases in Canada*, published by a branch of Canada Health and Welfare's Laboratory Centre for Disease Control, Dr. Bailar noted that "the long history of research that has focussed almost exclusively on treatment has not produced the benefits that we all hoped and expected to see."

Bailar wrote that he doubted a cure for cancer ever would be found. He described it as not one disease but many, each with its own characteristics. He suggested that it was time for a whole new approach, emphasizing prevention rather than treatment through a change in lifestyles and diet.

Said Chris: "Special interest groups, well-meaning as some of them are, seem to be responsible for much of the confusion over cancer treatment and results. Organizations that rely on public funding are inclined to suggest that donations are accomplishing more than they actually are. Sometimes to do this they put the best possible face on percentages and statistics."

She cited as an example a Canadian Cancer Society campaign slogan she had come across that promised "There's light at the end of the tunnel."

"From everything I'd been reading," Chris said, "I had to wonder what light? What tunnel?"

The big multinationals that manufacture the chemicals used in chemotherapy have a particularly good reason for putting a positive spin on success figures. This is a billion-dollar business. As long as chemotherapy remains in favor as one of the two major methods of treating cancer, these companies will go on making massive profits from the costly chemicals involved.

"Then there are the chemotherapists themselves," Chris said. "No one questions their belief in and dedication to what they do. At the same time, they have to give patients and their families potential success figures that belie a generally dismal record."

Just as oncologists progressively "stage" cancer to describe its severity, Chris came up with her own system of staging. It described her mental and emotional reaction to the disease from the outset. It, too, was progressive.

"Stage I," she said, "is the first and immediate stage that all cancer patients go through. You ask yourself, 'Why me?'

"Stage II is the acceptance stage: 'Well, whatever the reason, it *is* me!'"

Chris described Stage III as when you ask yourself "What am I going to do about it?"

"In the final stage, Stage IV," she said, "you develop an attitude: 'I'll be damned if I'm going to give in!'"

I knew the "Why me?" stage had been a traumatic time for my wife, as it is for everyone who has just been told they have cancer. There is a tendency to wonder if you somehow brought it on yourself. There is even the black thought that perhaps the disease is a punishment from God.

"What did I do that was so terrible," Chris wondered aloud, when she learned she had cancer, "that He did this to me?"

That may sound pretty strange, but it's a common first reaction among cancer patients. We threshed it out together one evening. Chris finally agreed that it made about as much sense as the idiot theory that God created AIDS to punish homosexuals.

The extensive research she did later told us that no one can say for sure what causes most types of cancer. Chris came to believe that lifestyle was a large factor in hers.

"We both know that I was always testing life to the limit," she said. "Doing so many things that were destructive of life, rather than supportive of it."

I had to admit this was true. Not just of Chris, but of both of us. I can't recall how often she dashed off to New York and Chicago to pick up awards for her work and put in exhaustive days cramming at week-long advertising seminars. Or how many times she worked through the night in television production studios in Toronto and Winnipeg editing commercials that always had to be in the can "yesterday."

"Always," as she put it, "running on overdrive. Smoking like a fiend. Eating fast foods, or high-fat restaurant meals with rich desserts."

Chris had decided early-on that genes also may have played a major part in giving her colon cancer. She read me the statistics—estimated, as always—that she had found.

"The average woman has just one chance in seventy of getting colon cancer. That escalates to one in two if two or more family members—grandmother, mother, aunt, or sister—also have it."

Chris's mother, Johan, was a remarkably strong-willed Highland Scot who had suffered for years from what she and her family referred to as "intestinal illness." When she finally agreed to an operation, she dropped to eighty-six pounds and was sent home from the hospital to die. That had been more than thirty years ago. She was now ninety-five. Her doctors called her "a survival miracle."

"Never once did she say the word 'cancer,' nor did she let anyone else in the family," said Chris. "Of course, that was what she had: colon cancer.

"I realize now that I inherited my mother's 'ostrich syndrome.' For all those years, knowing my mother had cancer, I had stuck my head in the sand.

"Even without knowing what I do now," she admitted, "I should have had routine examinations. The earlier a cancer's detected, the better the chance for longer survival. If some types are caught early enough, an actual cure may even be possible."

Chris had learned that this is important for anyone over forty. "It is absolutely essential," she said, "for someone with a history of cancer in the family."

Over the next while, she made her point in talks with her brother, sons, nephews, and nieces. Her message was simple: "Ask your doctor for a rectal examination when you get your annual check-up. If you feel chronically unwell in any part of your body, don't let your doctor give you a pat on the head and send you home with a pill. Insist that he or she carry out tests to find out why. Or find another doctor who will."

My wife had handled her own personal Stage II, her acceptance of her situation, by working hard at finding out all she could about cancer. This was her reality.

She moved on to her Stages III and IV—"What will I do about it?" and "I'll be damned if I'll give in!"—partly by taking a leaf from her mother's book.

"Mother beat the odds and stayed alive all those years," she said, "simply because she *willed* herself to live."

My wife didn't get any argument from me. Her mother had the kind of mind that does things you don't usually tell outside the family. Understandably, others would be sceptical.

I'll give you one example.

Some years ago, when our son Casey was just a toddler, he tipped a guest's cup of scalding hot black coffee onto himself. The skin of his chest came off with his undershirt. We rushed him to Emergency at Toronto's Sick Children's Hospital, where he was treated, bandaged, and released.

That same evening, we got a phone call from my wife's mother in Winnipeg. "What's wrong?" she demanded. "What's happened to my grandson?"

Over the years, there were other, similar manifestations of the unusual powers of this woman's mind. This led Chris to wonder if those powers had somehow helped her mother live for so long after she had been sent home to die.

Chris read a quotation she had recorded from the Chief Surgeon/Urologist (kidneys, bladder, prostate gland) at New York City's renowned Memorial Sloan-Kettering Cancer Center.

"'Mental attitude plays a larger role than we know in recovery.'" She quoted Dr. Willett Whitemore Jr. "'In some cases it might even make the difference between life and death.'

"This isn't a far-out theory by just one cancer authority," Chris said. "From what I've been reading, it's a belief from experience shared by a great many others."

I recalled her telling me, on the drive home from Polo Park Mall, what Dr. McIntyre had said: "Anger with your disease is good. But only if it's directed without, not within."

Chris suggested a comparison with "the guy who jumped for the high branch in Africa." She was referring to an item we had read some years earlier about someone who'd been chased by an angry rhino. It had made us chuckle, because it conjured up a serio-comic mental image as well as an interesting fact. Running for his life, the man had jumped for the high branch of a tree and made it. When he returned the next day and tried the same jump, he couldn't come close. His adrenalin rush, brought on by fear and a determination to survive, had given him the extra boost he needed.

"In a similar way," Chris said, "many oncologists believe that a cancer patient's anger with their disease, and will to live, may pump up their immune system."

As she so often did in these frequent talks we had, Chris came back to the concept of hope. It is, after all, the basis for all humankind's future. It is why we seek love and have children. It is the reason we get up every morning and that night look to a better tomorrow.

"Perhaps more than any other single thing," Chris said, "I'm beginning to believe it's what helps keep cancer patients alive."

She explained that she was speaking of realistic hope— "not the sort the spin-doctors hold out to make us feel better."

She had accepted her disease as probably chronic. One that could appear to be "cured," then recur at any time in the future.

She put it this way: "I tell myself 'Okay, so maybe I haven't won the war, but I've won the battle!'

"And if I can do it once, I can do it again. I can damn well win the next one! And if there's another, I'll win that one, too!"

Chris said that being told and believing she was "cured," only to have a recurrence of the disease at some point, would have desolated her.

"I'd rather look on it as my having won the first battle," she said with a sudden grin, "in what may turn out, I hope, to be The Hundred Years War!"

There were good times ahead.

I was still working on my dramatized biography of Dr. Charlotte Ross, which was taking much longer to complete than anyone had anticipated. Jack McClelland, who was then head of the Toronto publishing firm of McClelland and Stewart, had given me a six months time-frame in which to research and write a first draft.

Dr. Ross, who graduated in 1875 and was the first woman doctor to practise in Quebec and the Canadian West, had been all but lost in time. The answer to one question always led to several new questions. My wife and I had co-researched Dr. Ross and her family, in three countries and four provinces, for eight years. At one point, while I was still up to my eyeballs in microfilmed newspapers, Chris had been prowling around Winnipeg graveyards, thumbing through old records and checking headstones.

Now I had to correlate and interpret all that research so that I could accurately and with feeling tell this remarkable woman's life story. I spent my mornings bouncing up and down from my desk in a room literally papered with scotch-taped information slips. It was slow going.

With the comment "The game isn't worth the candle," Chris had given up the fast lane of retail advertising and promotion. She blamed her lifestyle and work habits, during her years in this career, as probably one of the reasons she had gotten colon cancer.

She now was seeking a more sensible way to live.

She looked for it in what, after her family, had always been her four principal interests: antiques, horses, purebred dogs, and cooking.

We seldom missed the monthly antique sales held by leading Winnipeg auctioneer Ron Peake and his wife. (One young girlfriend of our son Shawn's, visiting our house for the first time, exclaimed "It's like a museum!")

Chris had always liked the horses, primarily for the paddock parades and watching them run. We had visited Longchamps, where entire families enjoy an outing at the track, when we lived in Paris. In Toronto, we had been regulars at Old Woodbine, then at the New. Now, in Winnipeg, we were enjoying the occasional Sunday brunch buffet and playing the two-dollar wicket at Assiniboia Downs. Chris was a conservative bettor who carefully studied the Daily Racing Form the night before. She seldom won much, but she didn't lose much, either. I was a "hunch" bettor who won big once in a blue moon, but that was it. Usually, when I told Chris which horse I was betting and why, she just looked at me in disbelief and shook her head.

Chris and I always had loved dogs. For years we had bred, trained, and shown black Standard Poodles. Our champion pair—Beau Ideal and Ms. Liz—were from Toronto breeder Susan Radley Fraser's great international show and obedience champion, Bibelot Kennels' Tall, Dark and Handsome.

Chris did the hours of painstaking work required for each

show. She was the groomer, using all the tools and toiletries of a professional hairdresser and wearing a protective white smock. I was the handler, nattily dressed in navy blazer and grey flannels. She liked to tease about this among friends. "I do all the work," she'd say, "then the Glamor Boy, here"— indicating me—"runs around the ring a few times and gets the ribbons!"

The fact was, as everyone knew, I couldn't find the part in my own hair, let alone do a show job on a Standard Poodle's.

The fourth pastime that gave Chris great pleasure and at which she excelled was cooking and baking. Friends looked forward to her Saturday evening dinners for four.

It soon became clear that as well as Chris felt generally, the aftermath of her surgery made it impossible for her to continue grooming dogs. There was just too much standing and tedious hard work involved.

It's tough to explain to most people why anyone would put so much effort and expense into a few bits of ribbon, the generic trophies we called "Winged Victories," and a title for their dog. A good friend of ours, a golf fanatic, never could understand this. He finally urged us to get out of showing dogs and join his club.

When Chris demurred, and he asked her why, she replied: "Because I never saw a golf ball love you back!"

There is a spirit of camaraderie as well as competition among dog people. For years, wherever we happened to be living, Chris and I had played the regional circuits of weekend shows, usually within a day's driving distance. Like everyone else, we'd win some and lose some, working to "point" our dog to the title "Canadian champion." Then we'd meet and socialize with the other dog people at our motel, always beginning with a post-mortem on the day's judging. We had many good friends in dogs.

Reluctantly, we retired our Canadian Kennel Club breeder's registration, Bucko Kennels. "I'm going to miss the shows," Chris said.

"Well," I offered, "Beau and Ms. Liz are getting on in years anyway. Maybe it's time we all retired gracefully."

We only went to one or two shows after that. My wife, the consummate groomer and competitor, had no interest in being just a spectator.

Chris continued to have periodic tests, some of them at regular intervals. Every six months, she had to fast overnight and undergo a rectal examination by Arnold Rogers, with his periscope-like sigmoidoscope. He was looking for a recurrence of the small polyps, or tumors, that originally had led to her colon surgery. During one such examination, he found one and snipped it off.

I was waiting for her in the sitting-room at The Misery.

As we left the hospital, she told me about it, adding: "Rogers said it's not malignant."

My sigh of relief echoed her own.

I went with her to these twice-yearly tests by Arnold Rogers. While Chris always referred to them as "Another merry waltz with the sigmoidoscope!" I knew they were both painful and traumatic. She said she could take the lesser tests, like blood, X-ray, and general check-ups, on her own.

"You're sure?" I asked, biting my tongue. Worrying she might think I was being overprotective again.

She nodded vehemently. "Positive."

She didn't resent my concern. She simply had found a way to handle long waits alone in doctors' offices and testing labs.

"I know I identify with other patients," Chris said, "which sometimes has a scary effect on me. So I bring along a book and create my own space with a good read."

She explained that when she found the prospect of taking a test stressful, she worked at relaxing with deep, measured breathing. "Like the athletes do."

She also told me that she practised putting herself into "an altered state, a sort of trance."

"I let my mind take me to a happier, less complicated time and place. For me, it's always to the summers of my childhood, to the island cottage we called 'Ramona,' on Ontario's Lake of the Woods. It's comforting to be a young girl again, healthy and secure in family, with my father, mother, and two younger brothers."

This, she said, was one way she was learning to handle stressful situations. Another was to identify and talk with people. "Medical staff and technicians are human, too. They don't have my problem, but they've got problems of their own. I asked myself: 'How would you like to spend your day looking at one sad face after another and hearing nothing but complaints?' The answer came easy.

"So now I put on a cheery face, ask names, and strike up a conversation. Everybody likes to talk about themselves. If medical staff and technicians think you care about them, even casually, they'll be more inclined to care about you."

She said she had found that this helped both to reduce stress and to make her frequent lab tests less impersonal. "When you work at relating to people," she said, "It has a reciprocal effect. They begin to look upon you, too, as a person, which beats being just another number on a file."

This determination to remain a person, and to understand

and have personal input into her own health care, gave Chris a lot of problems.

When she gave one specialist a short list of questions about her treatment and its possible side effects, he glanced at it, tossed it back, and said: "I haven't got time for this. Why don't you go to Mayo?"

His reference was to the Mayo Comprehensive Cancer Center, the Mayo Clinic, Rochester, Minnesota.

His meaning was clear: If you want this kind of personal consideration, go where you get it by paying for it.

Chris found this to be one of the unfortunate spin-offs of our national health care system. "I call them 'the doctor-bureaucrats,'" she said. "They have the attitude that since the government pays the bills, we patients should sit still, keep our mouths shut, and do what we're told."

My wife and I, like a lot of other patients and their spouses, did a lot of just sitting.

When I was writing television plays in Toronto and Hollywood, Chris and I knew many young actors and actresses. They all hated what was known as "the cattle call." This is when a casting director puts out a blanket request for supporting actors and actresses. At the appointed time and place, dozens of young hopefuls show up to be looked over, interviewed and, with luck, offered a minor part.

I went with Chris to quite a few doctors' "cattle calls."

A dozen or more of us were told to show up all at the same time. We all did. We all sat and waited for the doctor's nurse to appear, read a name off her list, and say: "The Doctor will see you now."

As my wife's illness progressed and it became tougher for her to sit for long periods, we walked out on a few of these cattle calls. It was quite clear to both of us that as far as the doctor-bureaucrat is concerned, his time is important. Yours is not. Even though he may already have told you that you haven't got that much time left.

It became ludicrously apparent to both of us that some nurses practically deify their doctors. Once, after Chris had been kept waiting the better part of two hours, the nurse appeared with a beatific smile and said: "The *Good Doctor* will see you now."

Honest.

Not all of the doctors Chris saw were as elitist, or ran their office like some minor branch of government. She found that GPs, or General Practitioners, particularly those in family practice, generally had the best doctor-patient relationship.

"Probably because they relate professionally to the patient as a whole," Chris said, "and not just to that part of us that is sick, or diseased.

"Some doctors, specialists in particular," she said, "seem to lose sight of the patient-as-person and treat us as a case study. I'm not alone in this," she added. "I've talked with a lot of other cancer patients who feel exactly as I do: With many doctors, the disease, not the patient, is too often the focal point."

In my wife's continuing research into cancer and its treatment, she came across an interesting comment on this by Hippocrates. Hippocrates was the physician-philosopher who practised in Greece in the 5th Century B.C. To this day, his Hippocratic Oath is considered the equivalent of the Ten Commandments for the principled practice of medicine. Some doctors, I have noticed, have a framed copy hanging in their office.

"Hippocrates taught that it is just as important to know

the person who has the disease," Chris said, "as it is to know the disease the person has."

Not all of my wife's experiences, over her many battles and lengthy war with cancer, were like those I have just described. There were times when she, and the other cancer patients around her, received contrastingly personal and considerate treatment.

I was with her when she went for an appointment at the Tom Baker Cancer Centre, at Calgary's Foothills Hospital. This is one of the finest and most efficiently run cancer treatment facilities to be found anywhere. Appointments are individual and precise. When the interview with the patient preceding her took fifteen minutes or so longer than expected, a nurse approached us with a pleasant smile, an explanation and ("Would you believe that?!" Chris later exclaimed) an apology.

As well as this considerate staff attitude, the Tom Baker Cancer Centre provides an ambience that serves wonderfully to humanize it. Patients sit in one of a few small waiting-rooms off the main corridor. Each room is furnished like a sitting-room in your own home, with comfortable chairs, a large-screen television and a selection of current magazines.

Cheerful volunteers provide patients and those accompanying them with tea or coffee, served from pushcarts, in china cups and saucers. Cakes and cookies are home-baked by volunteers. Patients exchange pleasantries and chat, read, or watch tv. This and the relaxed, comfortable surroundings help create a less stressful, more pleasant experience.

Chris was impressed, as was I. "They should call it the 'Tom Baker *Caring* Cancer Centre,'" she said.

Since we weren't showing dogs any more, Chris spent more time in the kitchen. She was working on recipes and menus, low in fats and high in fibre, that she thought might be less likely to promote cancer. At about the same time, she came across cooking contests in two magazines, *Homemaker's* and *Western Living*.

As a cook-hobbyist, Chris always had imagined that more could be done with wild rice. The thought came naturally, since Lake Manitoba's Netley Marsh, just northwest of Winnipeg, is famous for its waterfowl and the wild rice they feed on. She often stuffed Cornish game hens with wild rice. Sometimes, for an off-beat and succulent vegetable dish, she mixed wild rice with Chinese snowpeas, water chestnuts, mushrooms and toasted slivered almonds. She decided to concoct a couple of new wild rice recipes to enter in the two magazine contests.

Our musician son, Shawn, was currently playing Winnipeg gigs. Chris began the trial and error process. Between us, Shawn and I ate so much wild rice soup over the next few weeks that we sometimes felt like we were drowning in Netley Marsh. This was followed by wild rice bread. Some of the recipes worked—almost. Some didn't. It was a great relief to both of us when Chris finally got them just right. Her "Netley Marsh Wild Rice Soup" and "Netley Marsh Wild Rice Bread" won a top-of-the-line food processor from *Homemaker's* and a hand-held electric mixer from *Western Living*.

She was having such a good time, she decided to go professional.

Everything about the "Baker Street Irregulars" was fun, beginning with the name, which she borrowed from Sir Arthur Conan Doyle's Sherlock Holmes fan clubs. She was a "Baker." She operated out of a private home on a "Street" in Winnipeg's residential River Heights. And this was "Irregular," to say the least. You could almost substitute "Illegal."

Within a couple of weeks, the Baker Street Irregulars was supplying specialty baking to a blue ribbon list of Winnipeg clubs: the historic Manitoba Club; the Winter Club; the Squash and Racquet Club; and the dining-room at Assiniboia Downs. She had started out with a state-of-the-art family kitchen. Now we went to a restaurant supplies auction and added another two stainless steel ovens and counter-tops.

I thought her stuff was a little pricy, but nobody complained. Everything from ingredients to execution was the best, and she did it all personally. Her "Queen Mum's" cakes, from a favorite recipe of the Queen Mother's, were garnished with real candied violet blossoms. When the executive chef at the Manitoba Club was sceptical that she used the actual French liqueur in her *"Gâteau Grand Marnier,"* and not just a flavoring agent, she included the empty bottle with his next order.

Chris was threatened by her own success on her first Christmas. She had discarded her recipe for the traditional, heavy English plum pudding with both a brandy sauce and a rich, hard sauce. She had found a lighter, much healthier one, that was served with a simple sherry sauce. The Winter Club ordered ten of them for a children's party. It was such a success that the chef rush-ordered another sixty to feature through the Christmas week.

"Sixty puddings!" I exclaimed. "Can you handle that?"

"No," Chris replied with a confident smile, "but I'm betting you can!"

Covering the dining-room table with a new painter's drop-cloth, I mixed, formed, bagged in cheesecloth, tied and steamed 120 pounds of Christmas pudding. For three full days, the kitchen was like a Turkish bath.

While the Manitoba Club required only a relative few for its much smaller membership, the puddings were a great success there, too. Chris got a call from the executive chef some months after she had gone into retirement. He asked if she'd bake again just long enough to provide the seasonal pies, cakes, and puddings that had been so popular the previous Christmas.

"What did you tell him?" I asked. Inasmuch as I was the Pudding Person, I wondered if I was going to have to haul out my painter's drop-cloth again.

"I said I was flattered," Chris said, "but no."

The baking had been very labor intensive. Chris had been finding over the past while that she was tiring more easily; that she had been having a gradual loss of stamina.

The Baker Street Irregulars never made much money. As a matter of fact, I think it was just a little better than a break-even proposition. As well as being a lot of hard work, it was expensive—the best ingredients came high. The important thing was that Chris had created a rewarding lifestyle for herself in her own way. She had found something challenging and worthwhile that she could still do, and she had had fun doing it.

There had been highs and lows, good times and sadness, in the two-and-a-half years that had passed since Chris's surgery.

We had lost Beau and Ms. Liz within months of each other. Our mischievous, loveable Ms. Liz had died following a major operation for a twisted intestine. Called gastric torsion, this is a fairly common and frequently fatal problem with some of the larger breeds. Our stout-hearted Beau reached canine senility. When I finally had to begin carrying him from the house out to the yard and back again, he begged me with his eyes to let him die with dignity. I owed him that. Our old friend went peacefully to sleep at the vet's, his head cradled in my lap, while I caressed that noble head and later wept.

Chris and I both realized we had to get another dog. The sooner the better. As western columnist for the Toronto-based national magazine *Dogs in Canada*, I had a reference library covering the 140-odd breeds recognized by the Canadian Kennel Club. Chris pored over these books for the better part of a week. Although she dearly loved Standard Poodles, she had decided she wanted a small dog that would be easier to groom and care for generally.

She finally chose the King Charles Spaniel. This is a toy breed, well-temperamented and weighing about twelve pounds, that has a great little sense of self. There also aren't many of them in Canada. We had to fly ours in from Christine Thaxton's Kings Court Kennels, in Chicago. Chris and Kings Court M'Lord Nigel hit it off the minute she hauled him out of his flight crate at Winnipeg International Airport. From that day on, they were next to inseparable. Nigel liked me okay, but he worshipped Chris.

The year following, Chris's mother died of a stroke at ninety-six. Even though this was a good old age, especially for someone who had been judged "terminal" more than thirty years earlier, it was a severe blow to my wife. She and her mother had always been very close.

Chris was a loving and considerate daughter. After a shaky start on both our parts, I, too, had grown to love this sometimes irascible, always resolute Scotswoman who was my mother-in-law. This should give you a small window on her character: I often heard Johan make the fey comment: "Life is very hard, and then you die."

One of Johan's favorite quotations was from the contemporary American poet Robert Frost: "The woods are lovely, dark and deep, but I have promises to keep, and miles to go before I sleep." When her mother died, Chris picked up on these lines as her own silent battle cry in her war against cancer.

During Johan's lengthy stay at Tuxedo Villa, Chris and I seldom missed visiting weekly with gifts of home baking, fresh fruit, or a small box of soft-centre chocolates or Turkish delight. Now and then we went for outings—a picnic at Assiniboine Park, or an evening cruise on the Red River on the *Paddlewheel Princess*. Sometimes we sat for a sherry in the Tuxedo Villa lounge, then had dinner together in the guest dining-room.

For some time after her surgery, these regular visits with her mother had been difficult for Chris. Using my Quebec shillelagh as a walking-stick, she had hobbled along the lengthy corridors; she had tried, for her mother's sake, to look better than she felt. Considering Johan's quick and intuitive mind, I don't think Chris fooled her even for a moment. But to the end, Johan clung to her unwritten rule: Not once in the two years following her daughter's surgery was the dreadful word "cancer" ever mentioned.

Chris had two nieces of whom she was very fond. They were sisters Debbie and Connie, daughters of her brother Don and his wife Pam. It had become a young family tradition for us to meet at Debbie's for a festive Christmas Eve buffet. Chris had baked a torte, seasonally blanketed with sliced red strawberries and green kiwis, as her contribution.

Early in the afternoon, Chris said she thought she'd lie down. Nigel, as always, followed her into the bedroom and jumped up beside her. After a while she got up and came back into the living-room.

"I don't think I can make it to Debbie's," she said.

I knew that my wife had been looking forward to this evening with her two favorite nieces and their families. She had spent that morning precisely slicing the fruit and putting the torte together.

"I just don't have the energy."

I was immediately concerned, but that was all. I had learned to know when Chris felt she needed her own space. I knew that if and when she wanted to talk about it she would.

We had planned to attend the annual Christmas Eve service at First Presbyterian Church before going on to Debbie's.

"What about the candlelight service?" I asked.

"I can still do that."

Chris was not a particularly religious person, but she and her family had occupied the same pew at First Presbyterian since she was a child. She had told me that sitting in that pew on occasional Sundays had made her feel closer to her Scottish-born father, who had died thirteen years earlier, and now it would make her feel close to her mother.

Quite apart from its religious significance, my wife was a fanatic about Christmas. She loved everything about it. We always had three trees at our house: the big one in the dining-room, which she always said was too small; a table-top flocked one in the living-room, decorated with precious little ornaments and called the "bird tree"; and another in the guest room.

All her life, Chris had been a child of Christmas. She had remained enraptured with the sounds, the smells, the spellbinding magic. Perhaps especially with the delicious business of exchanging gifts. I knew she had to be feeling seriously unwell to pass up going to Debbie's.

"You go," she said.

Did she really think I would leave her alone on Christmas Eve?

"I'll drop off the torte at Debbie's," I said firmly, "and tell her you're not feeling well. Then we'll go to the candlelight service."

The altar at First Presbyterian Church was ablaze with poinsettias. From the loft, the church choir carolled like angels. As though for the first time ever, the minister told the Christ Child story. As everyone lit and held candles in the dark, I glanced at Chris. She was caught up in the moment, as we all were. We exchanged a whispered "Merry Christmas!"

By hogmanay, the Scottish New Year, Chris was feeling much better. But not for long. Over the next two months, her energy ebbed and flowed at random, like an unruly tide.

On a Friday in mid-March, she had arranged to "do lunch" with Gerrie Morriss, an old friend and classmate from their school days. Chris hadn't been feeling sick. She had been eating well. But her energy had ebbed again and now she noticed that her stomach was swollen. She also was trace bleeding vaginally.

"You'd better phone Gerrie for me and cancel," she said. "I think I'd better phone McIntyre, too."

Chris didn't protest. I could see that she was hurting. She gingerly put a hand on her stomach. The swelling seemed more pronounced. She gave me a worried look. "I have a feeling something's terribly wrong," she said.

I got Don McIntyre at home.

"I don't think you have anything to worry about," he said, "but you'd better call Arnold Rogers, just in case."

When I reached Rogers, he listened to my description of my wife's condition and said, "Well, if you think she's sick, take her to Emergency."

There was no reason for either McIntyre or Rogers to re-act more positively than they did. Chris had been seeing both of them for regular check-ups. They knew that over a lengthy period of time she had been having good days and bad. This was not unusual for a cancer patient on a five-year "cure."

I phoned Emergency at The Misery and said I would be bringing my wife in shortly. We arrived just after 8:00 a.m. After being processed, given a hospital gown and checked over by the Emergency doctor, Chris was put on a gurney and parked on "gurney row" in the corridor.

It was a long day.

Don McIntyre and Arnold Rogers came by during their early morning rounds. Then Morris Broder showed up. It was three years to the month since he had done her colon surgery. He had Chris wheeled into an examining room and gave her a pelvic examination that she later described as "very painful." He left without comment.

Whatever problem she was having now, it hadn't dulled her appetite. About noon, she said she was starving and asked me to get her a "BLT," a toasted bacon, lettuce, and tomato sandwich, from the hospital cafeteria. I cleared it with the doctor in charge who, along with the head nurse, seemed surprised that Chris was even interested in food.

"It's her favorite sandwich," I explained lamely.

At about 10:00 p.m., Chris had a visit from the surgeon who is head of gynecology at The Misery.

"So now I have another doctor," she said. "He's an Irish-man named McCarthy. He gave me a 'pap smear.' I guess we're waiting for the results."

The pap test is given by collecting vaginal fluid. Intended primarily to detect cancer of the cervix, it sometimes may identify abnormal cells from other parts of a woman's reproductive system. In the hospital lab, a treated "smear" of the fluid is put on a glass slide. It is placed under a microscope and the cell structure read by pathologist. His findings are rated on a scale of 1 to 5. If it comes up as high as 4, it means there are enough abnormal cells present to do a biopsy.

Chris had been parked on "gurney row" for some fourteen hours. She grew reflective. "Just a while ago," she said, "I was sitting in the cat bird's seat. I was proud of my victory over cancer. I was having a lot of fun doing my baking. I was proud of myself and maybe a little smug. My mother had survived cancer. So would I." She shook her head. "I'm not so sure now."

This didn't sound like Chris. She was down, and I felt I had to say something to help bring her back up—even a little. I had told her that I would always be up front with her. I wasn't now. It's so easy to slip into a half-lie when you want so badly to shield someone. "Aren't you jumping the gun?" I said. "We don't know if it's all that serious."

Chris didn't bother to reply.

We both knew it was that serious. We were just waiting for someone to make it official. Chris had said early that morning that she had a feeling something was "terribly wrong." I wouldn't have phoned two doctors and checked her into Emergency if I hadn't felt she was right.

"I want you to go home and pack my 'happy bag.'" she said. "Bring a pillow, too, and my mohair blanket. And pick me up something to read—maybe the April *Vanity Fair*, if it's out yet. Otherwise, whatever."

She gave me a level look. "I'm not going to be getting out of here."

At about midnight, Dr. McCarthy returned to Emergency. He told Chris that she was being admitted for surgery.

Grandson Colin and "the bird tree." Christmas '89 — All her life, Chris had been a child of Christmas. She had remained enraptured with the sounds, the smells, the spellbinding magic.

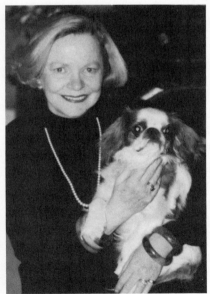

Chris and Kings Court M'Lord Nigel hit it off the minute she hauled him out of his flight crate at Winnipeg International Airport. From that day on, they were next to inseparable. Nigel liked me okay, but he worshipped Chris.

4 · Cancer strikes a second time

I should have known that Chris would not stay *down* for long.

She had passed sixteen hours or so in the hospital corridor, parked with other patients in the temporal purgatory of "gurney row." This, with anxiety over her condition, the tests she had undergone, and just being tired, had brought on her previous night's depression.

Early in the morning, I walked in to find the Chris I knew and loved.

"I want out of here," she said.

I liked her return of spirit, but I wondered if she had thought this thing through.

"What about the surgery?"

"I'll come back for that."

Dr. McIntyre had been in earlier during the course of his morning rounds. Ever since his respiratory arrest, and his own lengthy convalescence, he had developed an even greater empathy with his patients.

"Don McIntyre agrees that hospitals are no place for the sick if they can be at home. Especially on weekends."

It was a Saturday morning. Medical staff would be skeletal for the next forty-eight hours. Nothing would be done that could wait until Monday. McIntyre had arranged for Chris to get a weekend pass.

My wife got dressed. She had worn a shift. Loose-fitting as it was, I noticed it bulged at the lower abdomen.

Chris caught my eye. She laid a hand on her swollen dress and smiled self-consciously, "I feel like I'm pregnant again," she said.

In fact, it was the furthest possible thing from a blessed event. The swelling in my wife's lower abdomen was a tumor, a build-up of fluid resulting from her condition, or a combination of both.

She said her night nurse, whose name was Sonny, had gone to great lengths to help her rest comfortably overnight. She had not yet had time to establish a one-on-one relationship with the day nurse who arrived with the wheelchair. Her lower abdomen was so swollen, she had trouble getting seated.

At the floor station, the head nurse gave Chris her pass with a smile and an admonition: "We'll expect you back here Sunday night!"

As we wheeled down the corridor, Chris gave what amounted to a snort. "Where in the world," she asked of no one in particular, "would I go?"

Chris arrived home to an ecstatic welcome from Nigel. He was beside himself that she had not returned the previous night. He did what Chris called his "whirling dervish routine" in the entry hall. Then he settled down beside her on the living-room sofa while we talked over tea.

Dr. Gerard McCarthy had told Chris when he admitted her that he believed she had ovarian cancer. She got out her notes and we went over what she knew about this disease. Since her surgery three years earlier, she had researched cancers in general, and colon cancer in particular, but she didn't have that much information on ovarian.

What she did have was all bad.

"Ovarian cancer has been called 'the silent killer,'" Chris read from her notes. She indicated her swollen stomach with the page: "This is because it's difficult to diagnose until it has reached an advanced stage. The best way to try to catch it early is to have a pelvic examination once a year"—she glanced up—"like the one Dr. Broder gave me yesterday.

"And that," she concluded, obviously frustrated that she had so little, "is it."

Chris re-entered The Misery Sunday evening. Before I left her in the care of her night nurse, she made me promise to go to the library first thing Monday and read up on ovarian cancer.

This is what I found out: As is the case with most cancers, no one can say for sure what causes it. At greatest risk are women from age forty to sixty, and the risk peaks in the sixties. As with colon cancer, the risk rises sharply if two or more immediate family members—grandmother, mother, sister, aunt—have had ovarian cancer.

Since frequency of ovulation may be a factor, some oncologists believe that birth control pills may reduce the risk of getting this disease. So may having been a young mother, or a multiple mother. Oncologists are unsure whether it is the age at which a woman gives birth, or the number of times she does, that seems to reduce her chances of ovarian cancer.

Diets high in animal fats and low in fruit and vegetable fibres are suspect. So is talc, the principal ingredient in talcum and other cosmetic powders. Since talc often includes asbestos particles, a known cancer-causing agent, it is unwise to use these powders near the genitals, or on a diaphragm or condom.

The prognosis for ovarian cancer patients is not good. Most frequently, it already has had time to metastasize before it is detected. If it has spread to nearby lymph nodes, or surfaces of organs like the liver or intestine, it is Stage II. The "cure" rate, which means an extended five-year survival, is around 15 percent. At Stage IV, the cancer has spread outside the abdomen or invaded the liver. The five-year survival rate for this final stage is estimated at near zero.

Chris and I would not know what stage she was at until after her surgery, but it did not look good. She was showing growing signs of serious trouble. On the evening she had been re-admitted, she was fitted with an oxygen mask. She was having a problem breathing. Her bloating stomach was making it increasingly difficult for her to lie in bed. Her night nurse wheeled in a recliner chair from the corridor. With this ingenious maneuver, Sonny had managed to set Chris up in relative comfort.

McIntyre had said that hospitals are no place for the sick, if they can be at home. By extension, I felt that if Chris had to be in hospital, it should be as homelike as possible.

I loaded her makeup case with everything we thought she might need: mirror, brushes, combs, emery boards, Dove soap, perfumes, lotions, and cosmetics (but no nail polish!). In her closet were a warm wool robe and a lacy lounge one, a bed-jacket and nightgown, and unlike last time, pretty (but sensible) low-heeled slippers.

Our linen closet had provided two plump pillows with lace-trimmed slips. Folded at the foot of her bed was the fringed red mohair throw, woven in Scotland, that had been her mother's. The framed photo of us taken at the Banff Centre stood on her bedside table. Alongside were a designer box of Kleenex, the April *Vanity Fair* she had requested and Chris's newly discovered literary joy, *The Noel Coward Diaries*. Behind these was an arrangement of bright flowers in a heavy crystal vase that we had bought at one of Ron Peake's antique auctions.

"Home, sweet, home," Chris quipped from her recliner, but I knew she was pleased. Having some of her own things helped reinforce her sense of personal identity in an impersonal institution, however caring some of its staff might be. This piece of home away from home, this little corner of her life, did something else. It gave her the reassurance she needed that when they came for her for surgery, she had somewhere that was hers to come back to.

Chris had had one high point and a lot of low ones during her first few days in hospital after her colon surgery. She grinned when she described as a "high" point—"quite literally"—her encounter with quaint little Chaucerian folk who had come to visit her.

"I don't think I ever told you that I studied classic English authors at United College," she said. "A friend and I really got into Chaucer. For a while, just for the fun of it, we even spoke to each other in Middle English."

For a few days in the hospital after her colon surgery, Chris had been given morphine as a pain-killer.

"It created a lovely time for me," she said. "Little people from right out of *The Canterbury Tales* came and sat on the edge of my bed. They wore period costumes and chatted with me in Chaucerian English. For a while, they were delightful company." Then she added, a little wistfully, "But they left and never came back again."

The low points were caused by the staff cuts most hospitals have made, and continue to make, to save on operating costs. For the first few days of in-hospital convalescence after major surgery, some patients are helpless to do anything for themselves. Too frequently, there are too few nurses, trainees, and practical nurses to cope.

"You just have to spend a few days in hospital," Chris said, "to see that the nursing staff is generally understaffed and overworked. That doesn't help the patient who's in much pain and needs to change position, but can't. Or needs a mouth-wipe. Or is dying of thirst, and can only lie there and look at the water jug. Or who drops something and can't reach it."

We decided to hire a practical nurse for Chris's first few days after surgery. Neither of us was concerned with the standards maintained in the immediately post-operative Recovery Room, or Intensive Care. Don McIntyre had assured us, and we had seen from my wife's previous surgery, that when the level of nursing was critical, The Misery did not cut costs.

We were glad we had Blue Cross Extended Care Medical Insurance. Chris, the conservative horse-player who always played the odds, long ago had enrolled the whole family. I have to admit that had it been left up to me, I would have hunch-bet that none of us would ever get seriously ill!

Blue Cross Extended Care covered a lot of costs that regular health care didn't. Among them: A semi-private hospital room. The practical nurse Chris required, for three days and nights, on being returned to her room after surgery and Intensive Care. And later, a wig, when she lost tufts of her hair during chemotherapy.

She already had established first-name relationships over

her partial weekend and first full day in hospital. She spoke to me of Sonny, her night nurse, who so helpfully had hit on the idea of the recliner chair; Kelly, the station head nurse on days; and Sister Mary Anne, who visited the wards.

Days in The Misery begin and end with a prayer read over the PA system. Whether you are religious or not, and, if so, whatever religion you practise, is not relevant. The prayer always struck both Chris and me as being at once generic and oddly comforting. Throughout the day, sisters of the Oblates of Mary Immaculate visit and chat with patients, sharing in the high spirits of some, striving to lift the down spirits of others. Unless you want it to be, religion is not discussed.

"Sister Mary Anne has a great love of life and a wicked sense of humor!" Chris said. "I asked her about Dr. McCarthy. She told me he's head of gynecology here at The Misery, and a very good surgeon. She also said he's married, with about eight children—'though the Good Lord knows how, considering the hours he keeps!'"

Before the week was out, the sister and the surgeon, each in their own way, would do something caring for Chris that she found very touching. She would not know what this was, and tell me about it, until a few days after her surgery.

On her first full day in hospital, she was visited by Don McIntyre on his early morning rounds. Soon after, Arnold Rogers' approach was heralded by his stentorian voice and a round of laughter from the corridor. He entered with a retinue of young medical students.

Rogers sat on the edge of the bed. He took Chris by the hand and asked her how she was bearing up. He spoke to the students on the cause and effect of the swelling in her lower abdomen. He answered their questions.

"Then he made one of his typically Falstaffian exits," said Chris, "telling another of his jokes as he left." I have said that these two enjoyed each other. Now Chris smiled and shook her head. "I think Arnold Rogers always likes to leave his patients laughing!"

The seemingly endless, sometimes painful diagnostic tests on my wife began the next morning. Over the next few days, she was given blood work-ups, X-rays, ultrasound, and a pelvic sonogram—"and maybe a few others I lost track of," Chris said.

She was visited daily by a physiotherapist who coached her on how to avoid complications after her surgery. She got another piece of advice that led her to ask me to bring her a tennis ball. From previous experience, Chris knew she had "bad veins"—meaning hers were hard to find for blood tests and IV insertions.

"I mentioned this to an IV therapist on the day before my tests started," Chris said, "She warned me 'Never say you've got bad veins. They'll pick up on it and nine times out of ten it will go harder on you!'"

I had brought Chris the tennis ball she requested.

"The therapist told me I should get one of these and squeeze it for fifteen minutes or so a couple of times a day. She said this would help bring out the veins."

The pelvic sonogram had shown that the swelling in my wife's lower abdomen was being caused by a tumor and a build-up of fluid, called ascites. A chest X-ray had confirmed that this fluid had effused, or spread, to her chest cavity, pressing in on her lungs. Her difficulty breathing, because of this, had brought on the need for the oxygen mask.

On my next visit, I found Chris to be resting much more comfortably. She showed me her stomach, which was not nearly as swollen as it had been. In a procedure called aspirating, a needle at the end of a suction tube had been inserted between her ribs and fluid withdrawn.

Because the swelling was down and she was breathing a lot easier, so was I.

For the first time since he had had her admitted, at midnight the previous Friday, Dr. Gerard McCarthy dropped in on Chris. Again, it was late at night. She remembered what Sister Mary Anne had said about the hours he kept. Chris told me when I visited her the next morning how the meeting had gone.

"The Phantom Surgeon was here last night," she said.

She had me on that one. "Who?"

"Dr. McCarthy—the surgeon who's seldom seen, and then only late at night."

I had to grin. "Okay. What did you talk about?"

"He said he prefers late visits, what he calls 'the quiet times,' to speak with patients." Chris paused. "Sonny was here. When he asked her to leave, so we could talk privately, I knew this was going to be serious."

It was. They discussed the tests, the cancer and the surgery. McCarthy told Chris he thought she had a 30 percent chance of survival.

"I told him that I was expecting my first grandchild in June," Chris said; "that I had to live at least until then."

"What did he say?"

"He didn't. He just gave me a worried look."

Chris gave me a worried look of her own. "I know I'm in big trouble."

I was sitting on the edge of the bed. There wasn't much I could say. I certainly wasn't going to make the mistake again of trying to reassure her falsely with "We-don't-know-if-it's-all-that-serious." I took her hand in mine and because there was nothing to say, we just sat silent.

Chris was in more trouble than either of us realized. McCarthy had told her that he would be out of town for the next few days. He would do her surgery Friday. She asked him about this apparent lack of urgency, since there had been no time lost in getting her into hospital. He replied that there was still much prep to be done.

We found out the following day that this was only half the truth. A hospital panel has the final decision on surgery. Some doctors, including Don McIntyre, were not sure that it was the right way to go. While the ascites had been drained, and Chris could breathe freely and walk the hospital corridor at will, she was now known to have advanced cancer. Some members of her medical team were not convinced that she could survive major surgery.

The next day, Chris told me that McIntyre had come by earlier, on his morning rounds. He had explained the situation to her.

"He told me I had a choice," she said. "I could decide not to have the surgery. Whenever the ascites returned, I could have it aspirated again."

"What does Don think?"

She shook her head. "He said it's something I'll have to decide for myself. I don't much like the idea of just hoping the ascites won't build up again." She frowned. "It puts me in mind of the little Dutch boy who stuck his finger in the dike."

She said that Arnold Rogers had paid her a visit not long after McIntyre had left. This time he had come without a cluster of students.

"He didn't joke around like he usually does," Chris said.

"He just sat down and talked to me very quietly about my condition."

"And?" I prompted.

"He was very much to the point. He said 'If you were my wife, I'd want that thing out of there.'"

He was referring to the ovarian tumor, revealed by the pelvic sonogram, that had caused the ascites.

Rogers' comment may have been what made Chris decide to go for the surgery. It certainly helped. Having made that decision, she also make up her mind about something else. She decided if they wanted to see "healthy"—enough to okay the surgery—she'd *show* them "healthy!" She practised by the hour the deep-breathing technique her physiotherapist had taught her. She walked "miles of hospital corridor," as she put it, "squeezing on that damned tennis ball!"

"There was a positive side," she said. "I never had time to worry about the actual surgery. I was too worried they wouldn't do it."

The final and most critical test was for pulmonary, or lung, function. It would indicate whether Chris could breathe enough oxygen into her blood to help her survive the major surgery she faced. A physiotherapist explained that the procedure would be both lengthy and tiring. "Although it wasn't said in so many words," Chris told me later, "I got the impression that if I flunked out, there wouldn't be any surgery."

They came for her in a wheelchair.

"I knew that I had to pass this test. I had to think positive and work hard at it." This was what was going through her head as they wheeled her upstairs. When they got to where they tested lung function, it was explained to her that she would breathe pure oxygen. Then blood samples would be taken. "I was told that cooperation was very important; that I had to follow instructions exactly. I did. It was an ordeal, as the physiotherapist had said it would be. But when it was all over, I felt I had done well."

Chris wondered why Gerard McCarthy hadn't been around. Sister Mary Anne told her that he had flown to Manitoba's far north to operate on a seriously ill Native woman. Just returned that day, the Phantom Surgeon paid her one of his late night visits. Chris was right. She had done well. He told her the surgery was on.

Two anaesthetists came by to see Chris: one a day or so before her surgery, the other on the eve. The administration of general anaesthesia is a critical part of major surgery. This is particularly so for an older patient, or when lung function may be borderline. Listening to the second anaesthetist, Chris realized that the two disagreed on how to proceed.

She couldn't believe her ears. "So which will it be?" she asked.

"It depends on which of us comes up on the slate tomorrow," replied the anaesthetist.

"That was a real morale booster, the night before surgery," Chris said. So was the legal ploy that while she shouldn't let it worry her, she might get AIDS from transfused blood.

As it turned out, the wrong anaesthetist must have "come up on the slate." The anaesthetic he administered didn't hold her through to the end of her surgery. She came awake to excruciating pain—"as though someone were driving spikes into my stomach"—while they were still closing.

Chris had another late evening visitor shortly before her surgery. Dr. Robert Lotocki is a gynecologist oncologist. He explained that Dr. McCarthy had asked him to come by and speak with her. He asked me to stay while he discussed the follow-up treatment to my wife's surgery.

We found out later that Dr. Lotocki is on the cutting edge of the practice of chemotherapy. He told us that Chris should begin a series of eight treatments as soon as possible after her surgery. He explained that these would be given intravenously overnight, once about every four weeks.

"You'll have to change your lifestyle a little," Lotocki said, "to adjust to the side effects of the drugs." He briefly described some of these, such as weakness and nausea immediately following each treatment.

Later, when Chris began to read up on chemotherapy, we would learn that there were much more serious potential side effects. For the moment, though, in this room at The Misery, two days before her surgery, we were grateful to this obviously dedicated young specialist who had come to talk with us.

A couple of times while he spoke, Chris and I glanced at each other. She looked a little frightened and very confused. I figured that I probably did too. Neither of us had thought beyond her surgery. Now Chris had another critical choice to make, apparently almost immediately, about something of which we knew next to nothing.

"You're very fortunate," Lotocki was saying. "We're now working on clinical trials for ovarian cancer with a promising drug called Cisplatin." He went on to explain a little more about chemotherapy and the positive results they were having.

"If you were my mother or my wife," he remarked, as he moved to leave, "I would advise you to take these treatments."

The day before her surgery, Chris was given both blood plasma and antibiotics intravenously.

"The plasma IV was painful," she said later, "but I knew I had to be in the best shape possible. They started the antibiotic IV, to help prevent infections, early in the evening. It made me violently ill.

"With so many blood tests and IVs over the past week," she said, "I was glad for my tennis ball. I really think it helped!"

There was no discussion this time, as there had been before her colon surgery, about what to tell the boys. Shawn was already in town. I had phoned Rory and Casey a couple of days earlier. Casey and his wife, Elaine, walked in on Chris unannounced on the evening before her surgery. Without letting us know, they had booked a flight and flown in from Calgary earlier that day.

Although she had told me that she wanted the boys notified, but not alarmed, her face lit up like Christmas when they walked into the room.

"Casey! Elaine!" she cried out. "Where did you come from?"

"Calgary," Casey replied with a grin. He gave his mother a bear hug. "Where else?"

Elaine was holding a perfect red rose in a green glass bud vase. She put it on the bedside table, gently hugged Chris and kissed her on the cheek. Our daughter-in-law is by nature a gentle person. She also is a registered nurse who, at that time, was on the staff of Calgary General Hospital. She knew, and had told Casey, how critical his mother's situation was.

Chris had been keeping a detailed diary, both personal and medical, since just after her colon surgery, when she had begun her research on cancer. That night she wrote: "There never was a sweeter sight than Casey and my dear Elaine, pregnant with my first grandchild. I was truly thrilled to see them. But with my husband and Shawn already there, it emphasized for me the seriousness of the situation I was facing."

They came for my wife the following day just before 2:00 p.m., the scheduled time for her surgery. Casey and Elaine had spent the morning with her. I stayed on and we chatted about nothing. Kelly came in first, cheerfully efficient. Then the orderly. Chris helped them get her onto the gurney. I took her hand in mine, bent over and kissed her. "I'll be right here waiting for you," I said.

The young orderly obviously sought to raise the spirits of his gurney passengers, perhaps especially those bound for surgery. "We're on our way!" he sang out. He wheeled Chris out of the room. From the doorway, I watched after her down the long corridor and out of sight onto the elevator.

She told me later that one of the operating room nurses greeted her with a cheery "Hello!" Then he heard someone—she thought the anaesthetist—call out: "Where's Dr. Mc-Carthy?" Someone else answered, "He hasn't arrived yet." "Oh, God," Chris remembered thinking, "the Phantom Surgeon!"

A few minutes later, she was counting down to unconsciousness.

It was the racking pain of someone driving spikes into her stomach that brought her awake. She said later: "I wondered, 'Why is someone doing this to me?' I was still sufficiently 'under' that I couldn't focus on what was happening. I couldn't protest. As much as I wanted to, I couldn't even scream."

Chris came fully awake in Intensive Care. She was on IV. She was wearing a respirator that covered her nose and mouth. An electronic machine at her bedside monitored her life-signs. It was "beeping" to the linear breaks of an on-screen ball, familiar to anyone who has watched hospital drama on television.

I was standing by her bed. I was grateful that she had survived the surgery. I was also shocked by how pale and helpless she looked.

She told me later that the first thing her eyes had focussed on were the eyes of her nurse, a young woman of Oriental descent. Chris never got to know her name. She just remembered her as "Miss Gentle Brown Eyes." The nurse thought she wasn't warm enough. She covered her with a blanket and said "There, that's better."

When my wife's eyes found me, she managed to make them tell me that she was in much pain.

I looked across at the nurse. She had seen the look, too. "Can you give her something?" I asked.

"Miss Gentle Brown Eyes" shook her head. "I can't give her anything," she replied. "I'm afraid I'll lose her."

While Chris was unable to speak, or move, and was in great pain, she was fully aware. She heard and understood everything that was said by everyone around her.

"When I heard the nurse say that," Chris recalled, "I was really frightened. Then I gave myself 'a good finger-wagging!'"

This was an expression that she had picked up from the pages of *The Noel Coward Diaries*.

"I told myself: 'Okay, so you've lost control of your body. You've still got your mind. Make it make the rest of you live. Explain that you want to be a little old grey-haired lady, surrounded by grandchildren. Tell it not to listen to that dumb talk about somebody 'losing' you. Tell it you damned well won't *let* yourself be lost!'"

Chris was helped in her resolve by "Miss Gentle Brown Eyes" and the other nurses in Intensive Care. She later said that they showed a personal warmth and concern that went beyond medical professionalism.

She also said that she marked time between my visits, even though she could do little more, when I took her hand in mine, than communicate with her eyes. Her morale got a shot in the arm, too, from the phone messages she received from relatives and friends.

"The nurse would come and tell me that my cousins Ron and Don Gillies had phoned; or my dog-showing friend Vicki Feschuk; or Gerrie Morriss. Even though I could not speak with them personally, I looked upon all those thoughtful calls as rungs in my ladder to recovery."

Chris had undergone surgery on Friday. She made it out of Intensive Care, back to her own room, on Monday.

Susan, her private nurse, was there waiting for her. Except for brief coffee breaks, which she took only after first ensuring that Chris was comfortable, Susan and two other nurses worked round-the-clock shifts. They did this for my wife's first three days and nights out of Intensive Care.

"What a Godsend!" Chris said. "When I had to roll over, or needed a drink of water, or medication for pain, there was always someone there for me. On my second day, Susan rigged up a hair-washing apparatus while I still lay in bed. Clean hair was a miracle!" Chris was convinced that having her own nurse during those first few days had helped speed up her recovery.

I have mentioned that Sister Mary Anne and Dr. Gerard McCarthy—the sister and the surgeon—had done something personally very caring for her, each in their own way. It was just now that she learned what they had done.

Early on her first day back in her own room, Chris had a visit from the sister. After a brief chat, because she knew Chris would tire quickly, Sister Mary Anne moved to leave. She paused at the door.

"From when you were admitted," she said, "I prayed daily that your surgery would be successful. I thank God my prayers were answered!"

Soon after, an Operating Room nurse from my wife's surgical team dropped by to ask how she was doing. "It was touch-and-go for a while," she said. "Your blood pressure dropped dangerously low and you had dehydrated. Dr. McCarthy was very concerned. After the surgery, he sat by you in the Recovery Room. He didn't leave until he was satisfied that you were going to be okay."

"How long did he sit with me?" Chris asked.

"About two hours."

When my wife told me about these two vigils—one spiritual, the other medical—she added that she was very touched by both.

It was a day of visits. The next was from the physiotherapist who had coached her on how best to recover from her surgery. She already had begun kicking out with her legs, even before she had left Intensive Care. Now she was practising coughing. It was hard.

"As unladylike as this may sound," Chris said, "you hold onto your incision so you won't bust a gut. Then you cough." She demonstrated, wincing. "My entire insides hurt!" She had been told that this helps get rid of secretions in the lungs. "It's one of the most effective ways of avoiding post-operative complications," Chris quoted her physiotherapist. "Including pneumonia."

Her next visit was from Gerard McCarthy. "My Phantom

Surgeon had appeared briefly while I was still in Intensive Care," Chris said, "but I hadn't been able to carry on much of a conversation. Now I could, and I knew we had a lot to talk about."

McCarthy sank into the recliner at the foot of my wife's bed.

"He looked very grave," she told me later. "He wasn't at all his usual, cheerful Irish self."

Chris was immediately apprehensive. She took a deep breath. "Okay," she said, "what did you find? How did it go?"

McCarthy took a moment or two to reply. "I did a complete hysterectomy. Only one ovary was diseased, but I removed them both. I also did an appendectomy and an omentectomy."

The terms "hysterectomy" and "appendectomy" Chris understood. She later learned that an "omentectomy" is the removal of the omentum, a fat pad that hangs down from the large intestine.

"What happened to me in surgery?" she asked. "At some point I wasn't completely under."

"What do you remember?"

Chris told him about the awful feeling of spikes being hammered into her stomach.

"You don't remember that."

"Oh, yes, I do! How could I ever forget!"

McCarthy didn't reply. It was a few days later that what Chris remembered so vividly was confirmed as not just some anaesthetically induced nightmare. "Near the end, I knew you weren't completely under," another member of her surgical team told her. "Your eyes were open."

We learned much later that what Chris had suffered through is not an uncommon experience. There are hundreds of such cases in the files of an American association called Awareness, which is based in Virginia. In each case, a patient who had been given the wrong anaesthetic, or not enough of the right one, had come fully awake, or "aware," in the late stages of their surgery. All reported being panicked by excruciating pain and frustration. Though they were fully conscious of what was happening to them, the anaesthetic had kept them powerless to do anything about it. Even to cry out.

My wife had a lot of pain in the days immediately following her surgery. Said one of her nurses, matter-of-factly: "You don't get brownie points for suffering. If you don't need the medication I just brought you, leave it until you do. Then take it as soon as you start to hurt. It's better to chase the pain than have the pain chase you!"

Her physiotherapist visited daily to listen to her cough. Chris apparently was one of her prize patients. "Dry as the Sahara!" she would exclaim, waxing almost poetic over my wife's suitably arid lungs. Then, hurrying off to check on her next hacker, "Keep up the good work!"

Chris coughed well. From when she first started feebly kicking out in Intensive Care, she did everything she was asked to do. "Whatever it takes to go home," she said.

As she had after her colon surgery, she walked the corridors with her "boyfriend," pulling the wheeled IV along with her a little further every day. While exercising to get her strength back physically, she worked at *willing* herself well again.

Both determined efforts were not without their setbacks.

A few times in the beginning, she overdid the walks with her "boyfriend" and had to cut back on distance over the next day or two. About a week into her recovery, our youngest son, Shawn, and I were visiting. We three were chatting about nothing in particular. Chris appeared to be in good spirits. Abruptly, her whole manner changed. Her face crumpled and she burst into tears.

She told me later that she had never seen my look so stricken. I could believe that. While Shawn stood confused, I hurried out to the Nursing Station. Kelly was on duty. By the time we got back to the room, Chris was dabbing at her eyes with a clutch of tissues Shawn had given her. As quickly as she had lost it, she had composed herself.

Her teary-eyed smile was embarrassed. "I'm sorry."

I went and embraced her, while Kelly fussed with the IV at her bedside. "For God's sake," I said, "you don't have anything to be sorry *for!*"

Kelly had told me as we strode from the Nursing Station to my wife's room that her sudden, emotional outburst was perfectly normal.

It was the psychological as well as the physical impact of her total hysterectomy. Perhaps even more traumatizing, Kelly said, she had come to realize, finally, how very seriously ill she was with cancer.

If we had any wishful doubts about that, they were quickly dispelled over the next few days.

"The Phantom Surgeon comes by every night," Chris said. "He talks to me about my taking chemotherapy." She paused. "Whether I do or not, my prognosis isn't all that great. But he says chemotherapy might give me—us—more time."

My wife was being asked to make what could be life-or-death decisions, just days after she had barely survived surgery. I felt like saying "It's so damned unfair!"

Instead I said "How much time are we talking about?"

"A year maybe. McCarthy seems to think longer, if I take chemotherapy. He's being very straight. He admits there's actually no way of knowing."

"Have you decided?"

Chris shook her head. "I want some answers to some questions first." She tossed a few at me. "Are they really sure it will do any good? How damaging are the side effects? How sick will I get?"

Then she added quietly, "More important to me than anything, more important than life itself, is the quality of my life."

Quality of life.

What a simple phrase it is! I did not realize then how charged with meaning it would become for both of us. How greatly it would dictate my wife's decisions on cancer treatment. How much it would affect the rest of our lives together.

Right then, though, I just figured that Chris needed a lift, even if only a small one.

Her loyal and little friend Nigel is a compact twelve pounds. On my next visit, I tucked him out of sight inside my trenchcoat and strode casually across the hospital lobby. Immediate family members of critically ill patients and new mothers are allowed off-hours visits. A uniformed security guard was checking passes at the elevators. I already had mine in my free hand. He nodded acknowledgement and I filed past him with several other visitors.

I was not concerned with Nigel giving us away. His breed is the canine soul of propriety. Chris used to say that if the whole world were populated by King Charles Spaniels, instead of people, we would not need police, armies, or the U.N.

They can, however, be innocently curious.

Just below my wife's floor, Nigel poked his head out the

flap of my trenchcoat. The breed is pug-nosed and long-eared, with soft, button eyes and a fluffy fur coat. They look as much like a stuffed toy as a real live dog.

A woman glanced our way and smiled benignly. I could read her mind: *Someone on his way to visit a sick child? A precocious gift, perhaps, for a new-born baby?*

Her eyes widened when Nigel's head moved.

"Gund," I said, naming the famous stuffed-toy maker as I stepped off the elevator. "Remarkably lifelike."

Behind the closed door to her room, Chris was hugging Nigel and laughing her pleasure at his frantic attempts to hug her back. She flashed me an amused look over his bobbing brown and white head. "You fool!" she said.

By now, Chris had the feeling that she was being campaigned, not just advised, to take chemotherapy. Even Kelly, her head nurse, was urging her to go for it. Dr. McCarthy said that he would like to transfer her the following week from The Misery to St. Boniface Hospital—"St. B."—in the city of that name, just across the Red River from Winnipeg, for her first treatment.

I asked her what her reply had been.

"I was shocked!" she said. "I think I said something that showed it, like 'You must be kidding!'" Then she had added "My God, I haven't had my stitches out!"

McCarthy had ignored this. "The sooner chemotherapy is started," he had said, "the better your chances are."

Chris had dug in her heels. "I don't care. I need some time. I need to know what I'm getting into. I haven't even seen a report on my surgery!"

While it may not sit well with some members of the medical profession, the patient's "right-to-know" has been upheld by the courts. This includes access to all medical reports and hospital records that relate to the patient personally.

Chris asked to see her surgical report. It was brought without comment and dropped on her bedside table. Whether from professional pique or simple thoughtlessness, no one offered to help her with it. Telling me this brought a puzzled frown to her face. "It only would have taken a minute or two," she said. Characteristically, she abruptly grinned. "For the most part, that report might as well have been written in Swahili!" What little she did understand had disturbed her. She had written down the rest and asked me to use the medical dictionary at the library to decipher it.

Beyond the fact that Chris had undergone a total hysterectomy, which we already knew, we learned from the report that her cancer was Stage IV. This is the final stage. It means that malignant cells have spread to random parts of the body and the patient has advanced cancer. It can't get any worse.

Disturbingly, the biopsy could not conclude whether her tumor was a "primary" or a "secondary."

Simply put, if her tumor was a "primary," it had originated in the ovaries and she had ovarian cancer. If it was a "secondary," her first cancer had metastasized. This meant that she did not have ovarian cancer, but that her colon cancer had spread to the ovaries.

This is what finally decided her to put off chemotherapy until she had more time to learn and think about it. The chemo for colon cancer is different from the one for ovarian. Which would they choose? Would they make the right choice? And who'd ever know for sure?

When Kelly came into the room, Chris was dressed and putting the last of her things into her "happy bag."

"Dr. McCarthy didn't say anything about you going home today . . . "

Chris smiled angelically at the head nurse. "I was told by a very smart doctor that a hospital is no place for the sick, if they can be at home. I phoned my husband. He's coming for me at noon. We've got a date to watch the Academy Awards."

Kelly hesitated. "I'll check with Dr. McCarthy," she said.

When McCarthy arrived, he was a little miffed that Chris had decided on her own to leave the hospital. Then, knowing her as he did, I guess he realized that it was something he should have expected. He satisfied himself that she would be well cared for at home. He cautioned her not to overdo it. Then, before he signed her release, he said he hoped she would seriously consider chemotherapy.

From what Chris told me, the Irish surgeon and the Scottish patient had developed a wary sort of friendship during their nocturnal talks about Celts, Gaels, cancer and chemo. She had thanked him earlier for his two-hour vigil in Intensive Care, telling him how touched she had been. Chris said later that he had looked a little embarrassed. The Phantom Surgeon wasn't aware she had known about that.

Always the conservative horse-player who read the form sheet and played the odds, Chris went one-two-three in her Academy Awards selections. We did our annual Awards-watch in the living-room, where I had made up a sofa-bed. I had to endure an evening of "I-told-you-so's!" as she scored with *The Emperor* for Best Picture, *Moonstruck*'s Cher for Best Actress, and *Wall Street*'s Michael Douglas for Best Actor.

Next on her agenda, Chris would do her level best to work out the odds on chemotherapy.

5 · "The Chemistry Boys"

"I guess it's appropriate that both words are from the Greek," Chris said. She was referring to "oncology" and "hedonism."

The Greeks gave us the root word for "oncology," which is the study and treatment of cancer. They also gave us "hedonism," which loosely translates as eat, drink, and be merry. This was the one word of advice that Dr. McIntyre gave Chris on his first house call after her surgery. She was sitting in a little room off our bedroom that we had converted from what had once been a back porch. It was a sunny retreat, brightly papered in blue and white flowers-and-stripes and furnished with antique white wicker that had come from "Ramona," the family cottage at Lake of the Woods. Chris had made the yellow plaid cushions for the two chairs herself.

Dr. McIntyre arrived early and unannounced. I showed him into the back room. Chris didn't have to say how delighted she was to see him. It was written all over her face. He was our friend, as well as Chris's primary physician. She had told me just the night before: "If there is one doctor I can trust to tell me the truth, it's Don McIntyre."

There is one question that cancer patients desperately want answered, but often are afraid to ask. After the usual pleasantries, Chris put it to Don McIntyre point blank.

"How long have I got?"

It seemed an age before he answered.

"A year," he said. "Perhaps a little longer."

There was a lengthy silence. The expression on my wife's face clearly said *Well, I asked for it!*

"What if I take chemotherapy?"

McIntyre again took his time before replying. "I wouldn't count too much on it."

Both Chris and I knew that he was not gung-ho on chemo. At one point he had even asked "Are those guys"—not bothering to identify who 'those guys' were—"pressuring you to take chemo?"

Chris had said he seemed to be the only one who was listening when she spoke about quality of life. Now he offered his advice on how best to handle her disease and get the most from whatever time she had left.

"Hedonism," he said. "Get the most pleasure you can out of every new day."

In the weeks, months and years to come, these became key words in Chris's definition of quality of life.

Leaning on my Quebec shillelagh and hobbling about the library wasn't the most pleasurable way for Chris to spend the next several days. When I pointed this out, expressing my concern that she was not that long out of surgery, she said "I don't have a choice. I'm not going to be led blindly into chemotherapy or be steered away from it. It's something I'll decide for myself. I can't do that without finding out as much as I can about it."

We met at noon in the library lunchroom. Over my

lengthy research on Dr. Charlotte Ross, and Chris's on cancer, we had developed a nodding acquaintance with the staff. The woman behind the sandwich and salad counter smiled hello and asked Chris where she'd been. This happened often. My wife was an easy person to remember.

Have I said she was beautiful? I thought so from the moment I first saw her, typing newspaper copy at a desk halfway across the editorial room from me. I thought so now, thirty-seven years later. She had had her hair done a few days earlier by Mario. She looked good and she looked well.

Chris had tried various cosmetic products to camouflage post-surgery pallor and to use on those days when the cancer within showed through and made her pale. She found that Estée Lauder's Self-Action Tanning Cream gave her face a natural, healthy look. She also had satisfied herself, through a professional cosmetician, that it contained no possible cancer-causing ingredients.

Before she finished removing the plastic wrap from her salad, Chris began telling me what she had learned about chemo. She frowned her frustration.

"Like everything else about this disease," she said, "it's all so damned inconclusive! Chemo is known to slow down the spread of some cancers. Even effect an actual cure in a few. But not with most." Her frown deepened. "And there are so many differences of opinion."

Chris gave her own situation as an example. A few days earlier, an oncologist she had consulted for a second opinion had told her that without chemotherapy she likely had only months to live. That morning in the library, she had made a note of this quotation from an eminent American oncologist: "Fifty percent of women with ovarian cancer fail to respond to chemotherapy."

"I'm also disturbed by the 'chemo'—the poisonous chemicals—in 'chemotherapy,'" Chris said. "They're meant to kill, or slow the growth of cancer cells, or shrink tumors. The problem is that they also poison the healthy cells.

"The treatment is stopped before the damage done to the patient's immune system is irreparable. Because the healthy cells recover faster than the diseased ones, the patient is ready for another chemo session within a month or so."

The use of chemicals to combat cancer sprang from the deadly "mustard gas" that the Germans released without warning in World War I. Specific effects on devastated Allied troops led to the development of chemotherapy by American researchers in the 1940s.

I was pretty sure how I would feel about what amounted to poisoning my own immune system. I wondered how Chris felt.

"I think it's obscene," she said.

She paused thoughtfully before adding "Then there are the side effects."

Chris read from her notes: "Depending on the chemo you are given, these can be anything from impotence and sterility to mental problems and new primary cancers."

She admitted that those were "the worst possible scenarios."

She described more likely side effects as the lessening of the body's ability to fight disease, through suppression of its white cells. Intense nausea. Hair loss. And chronic depression.

"There also is the possibility that after the first few treatments, the cancer cells will develop their own immune system to resist the drugs being used.

"It all seems very 'iffy,'" Chris concluded. "And after all

that, when you've finished your series of chemo treatments, it's back to surgery so the Chemistry Boys can 'go in for a little look.'"

This was the expression Dr. Robert Lotocki had used when he spoke to us that night in the hospital, while Chris was awaiting surgery. It is the usual follow-up procedure to ovarian chemotherapy.

"'Go in for a little look!'" Chris had parroted after his departure, not without some humor. "The next time I see that man, I must tell him that I am not a shoe box!"

I could see that someone was going to have to do some major convincing to get my wife to agree to chemotherapy. It would not be me. We had laid the ground rules much earlier in the game.

It was her cancer. She appreciated, even constantly asked for, my opinion, my input. But that was all. When the discussions with the professionals and between ourselves were done, it came down to rights and responsibilities. It was her right to decide. It was my responsibility to support her in whatever decision she made. It was her life.

Just about everyone knows someone who has cancer, or is close to someone with the disease—a family member, relative, or a friend. As well as reading up on it at the library, Chris and I spoke with people who had taken chemo, or knew someone who had.

Our findings could not be considered anything remotely resembling a study. But they did give her a glimpse of the human face of chemotherapy, behind the computerized statistics and percentages.

What we learned in these conversations was not encouraging. Some cancer patients had died before they had finished their series of treatments. Others had died soon after.

Still others had died some months or some few years later. Summing it all up, as far as Chris was concerned, was the post-operative lifespan of two brothers in Winnipeg, each of whom had made his own decision on whether or not to take chemo.

"One had gone for it, the other hadn't." she related. "I was told by a family friend that both had died within a few months of each other."

Despite all the negatives that Chris had turned up, it didn't change the fact that conventional medicine is committed to chemotherapy. This presented her with an ongoing dilemma.

We had received phone calls from Dr. McCarthy and Dr. Lotocki. Both wanted to re-impress on Chris that if she were going to take the treatments, it was vital that she begin as soon as possible after surgery.

"God help me!" she said at one point—not as an expletive; more like she was asking Him for guidance. "I'm afraid to take chemo and I'm afraid not to!"

What finally tipped the scales was the suggestion by Dr. McIntyre that she give it a try. This was something of an about-face for him. It resulted from a discussion of my wife's condition with a colleague, an oncologist whom he had known and respected for years.

Lotocki had told Chris she would be given eight treatments, one about every four weeks over eight months.

"Try one or two and see how it goes," McIntyre counselled. "Nothing is written in stone."

Chris had heard that expression from a member of her medical team before. At one point, she had gotten the impression that if she did not agree to follow-up chemotherapy, she might not get the surgery she needed.

"Nothing was ever said by anyone," Chris later told me. "It was just a feeling I had.

"It was in the hospital, while I was awaiting the decision on my surgery, that I mentioned this to Arnold Rogers. He said the same thing Don McIntyre said: 'Nothing is written in stone.' That was all. Then he turned and left the room."

It was just a few days after Dr. McIntyre suggested that Chris give chemotherapy a try that we met with Dr. Lotocki at St. Boniface Hospital. We had an early morning appointment. We sat with a number of other patients in the Oncology waiting-room. Lotocki's nurse, Bernice, periodically emerged from a corridor of offices and called out a patient's name.

It was a somber group. Most of the men and women sat in silence, or spoke with companions in the hushed tones that people use in church. A couple of men wore toque-like caps, obviously to cover their hair loss, called alopecia, which is a side effect to some types of chemo. A woman had a tam pulled down to her ears. Another wore a sort of turban. There was a self-serve kitchenette, offering coffee in styrofoam cups, powdered creamer, and Christie's biscuits.

When Chris was called, Lotocki discussed her chemotherapy with her. Then he told Bernice to arrange for immediate pre-chemo assessment, which included blood tests and X-rays. She was to be admitted for her first treatment the next day.

I didn't dare look at Chris.

The next day, April 15, was her birthday.

I knew what she was thinking.

Some birthday present!

From Chris's notes, we knew that there are several ways to administer chemotherapy, including orally and intravenously, and many different drugs. It depends on the type of cancer and the stage it has reached. The treatments do not come pre-packaged with directions and dosage. Often drugs are used in combination, customized by the chemotherapist for each individual patient. The patient's responses are carefully monitored by blood work-ups between treatments.

"Obviously," Chris concluded, "you should choose a chemotherapist as carefully as you would a surgeon."

On that day before she began her treatments, Chris told me that she had full confidence in Robert Lotocki as a chemotherapist. Her only misgivings were about chemotherapy itself.

By the time Chris's pre-chemo assessment was finished, there was a new batch of people seated in the waiting-room. We both noticed that the atmosphere was just as glum as before.

"How can this be positive," Chris asked as we stepped outside, "when everyone looks so negative?"

Because her cancer had been diagnosed as advance ovarian, Chris was to be given a combination of two drugs intravenously: Cisplatin and Cytoxin. She had read that, due to their extreme toxicity, these two have been called "the gold standard" of chemotherapy drugs.

"The toxicity of other drugs," she elaborated, "are measured up to them."

Neither of us spoke for most of the hop, skip, and a jump over the Red River that gets you from St. Boniface into Winnipeg. Chris finally broke the silence. "Lotocki said that much of the nausea associated with chemo may be mental. He's known of patients who begin feeling sick on the drive to the hospital."

Chris had learned that some patients suffer less nausea from chemo if they smoke marijuana. Lotocki had told her that the responsible ingredient was available as suppositories. She also had read that patients could get actual marijuana legally, by prescription. "Though this may be just in the United States," she said.

If this were so, it didn't matter. We didn't pursue whether you also could get it by prescription in Canada. The report Chris read counselled that it's better to get it on your own.

"Apparently the stuff on the street," she said, "is better than the stuff from the government."

The same report pointed out that marijuana helps combat chemo-induced nausea in some patients, but not all. Chris and I agreed that it was worth a try.

We knew that getting it wouldn't pose much of a problem. Shawn's band was playing the Northwestern Ontario-Manitoba circuit, but they were currently in Winnipeg. Even if he didn't smoke the odd joint himself (God forbid!), his mother and I figured that he might have a musician friend or two who did.

We celebrated Chris's birthday with one of her favorite dinners, served early because she had to check into "St. B" by 7:30 p.m. The entrée was fresh fillet of sole, lightly floured and browned in a small amount of butter, garnished with parsley and served with a lemon slice. The wine was an '82 *Pouilly Fuisse*. The cake, from the Belgian Pastry Shop, had only symbolic candles, something decreed by Chris some years earlier, when the actual count had reached thirty. One of her gifts was a dozen slim, hand-rolled cigarettes, twisted at both ends. Shawn advised her to wrap and store in the freezer those she planned to keep for next time.

"When do you smoke these?" I asked Chris.

"I don't know," she confessed. "I guess I'll have one before we leave for 'St. B.' Then after that 'as required,' as they say."

She slipped a few into her purse, while I went for the "happy bag." We had packed it with just the few things that she would need for an overnight stay. She had added a remarkably powerful, pocket-sized Sony AM/shortwave radio that Casey and Elaine had given her. On nights when worry kept her awake, she enjoyed listening to Larry King, Sally Jessie Raphael, and the broadcast Tower of Babel that is shortwave radio.

She also had packed a satin pillowcase. When she started losing her hair, the slick satin would not pull at it like a cotton one would, making her lose more of her hair faster.

Because Chris had quit smoking some years earlier, she resented having to smoke the marijuana cigarette. She also didn't like the taste. Driving her to the hospital, I was curious to see if she would get a little giggly. Nothing. I hoped it would have more effect on the nausea.

We were almost there when something struck me as funny. "If the police stop us and check your purse," I said, "we'll both be up on drug charges."

Chris rolled her eyes. "Drive carefully," she said.

My wife checked in at the nurses' station and was given a room number. She was told that a nurse would be along shortly. We followed the numbers down the hall, came to the right room, and entered. Chris and I looked at each other. I saw her heart sink. It was a small room with two beds that could be partitioned off with the usual hospital curtain. The paint on the faded green walls was peeling in places. The bathroom fixtures were antique without the charm.

I was shocked and I could see that Chris was, too.

"This would make a room in the Tower of London look like Happyland," she murmured.

We talked about it later. "St. B." is a historic Manitoba hospital with old and new sections. You can't fault it for showing its age in places. But we both felt that something should have been done, even if it were only cosmetic, to help lift the spirits of patients taking chemotherapy. To brighten their surroundings. To boost their morale. To make them feel a little special. Lord knows they deserve it. I thought of petitioning the Hospital Board for something as basic as a can of paint before Chris and her chemo partner had to return for their next treatment.

Whoever was to be her roommate hadn't arrived yet. A pleasant young nurse entered the room and introduced herself as Tannis. She gave Chris an encouraging smile and a hospital gown and went away again.

Chris got settled into bed with *Vanity Fair*, her radio, and bottle of Perrier on her bedside table. Her blonde hair lay against the pink satin pillowcase. "Well," she said, "my first time for chemo."

"How do you feel?" I asked.

"Like *The Reluctant Debutante*," said Chris, quoting the title of a Rex Harrison-Kay Kendall romantic comedy that we'd seen a few nights ago on the Late Show.

If she could joke about it, I figured she was going to be okay. I bent down and kissed her goodnight.

When I came for Chris about noon the next day, she looked pale and shaky. So did her roommate, a woman of about the same age. As soon as I got Chris home, she went to bed. She looked and felt miserable. She had diarrhea. She threw up that day and into the night. When there was nothing left to throw, she had the dry heaves.

She also had considerable pain in both her colon and groin. The pain in her chest for the first day or two, she attributed to anxiety. Her hurting and being generally unwell lasted for about a week. Her brother Don brought her a cordless phone so she could make and receive calls in bed. The worst part was that all I could do was sit and watch. There was absolutely nothing I could do to help.

For some time after Chris and I learned she had cancer, we had to struggle through a great deal of confused anger and guilt. She was angry that she had been stricken. I was even angrier, if that were possible. She felt guilty that she had somehow brought it on herself. I felt guilty that Chris had gotten cancer, instead of me. With someone you love, I am told, these feelings of anger, guilt, and frustration are normal.

Now, watching her suffer the side effects of chemotherapy, I blamed myself more personally.

I had agreed with her that she should try it. Maybe, because I hadn't opposed it, I had been partly responsible for her decision. I had driven her to the hospital. I had left her there to be carefully poisoned.

I wondered if I could have been a better friend.

The side effects Chris was experiencing seemed to be cumulative. She reacted even more badly and for a longer period of time to her second chemo, which she was given twenty-eight days after the first.

The marijuana cigarettes didn't help. She had read that they worked for some people, but not others. "I guess I'm one of the 'others,'" she said. Months later, looking for cookies Chris might have stashed away, I was squirreling around in the freezer after she had gone to bed and found what was left of the cigarettes in a plastic pouch. I had never smoked marijuana. Sitting alone, watching the Late Show, I tried one. It didn't do anything for me, either.

When Chris watched television, she was back to squeezing the tennis ball I had brought her when she was in The Misery. It was helping to bring out the vein in the arm in which they inserted the IV needle for her chemotherapy. First one hand, then the other. Four hundred times each, daily.

She was using a lot of Self-Action Tanning Cream to cover what had become chronic pallor, lasting for about two weeks after each treatment. She had always valued her appearance. Now she worked even harder at it. "If you look good," she said, "you'll feel good; or if not good, at least a little better." Her hair had been medium length. Her hairdresser advised her to let him cut it short.

Mario had counselled other clients who had taken chemotherapy.

"He told me hair is easier to handle when it's short, and a wig fits better," Chris said. Mario ordered the wig for her. "A good synthetic that I can just wash and shake dry. Lightweight and on a net base so it won't be too hot in summer."

Mario's professional hairdressing trick was to customize the wig; to shape it to her head. Which is what he did. I had to agree with Chris that it looked remarkably natural. As well, she liked her new short hairstyle so much that she kept it after she was finished with chemotherapy.

As negative as the reason was for the wig, my wife, in her typical way, found a positive side. "When I'm done with chemo," she said, "it will come in handy for after swimming."

Chris had been told that she wouldn't start losing her hair until after her third treatment. Even though she washed her hair gently and used a conditioner, as Mario had suggested, her hair began coming out in tufts after the second. Her feeling of extreme fatigue and being generally unwell lasted ten days. For most of that time, Chris lay in bed.

"Even when I'm well enough to be up and around," she said, "I feel blown away. What bothers me most is that chemo seems to erode the will. At least, it does with me." Her tone had been tentative. Now it became determined. "I can't let that happen. I know that when I lose my will to live, that is when I will die."

She lost her appetite to chronic nausea, and the mouth sores brought on by chemo that made it painful for her to eat. She ate on whim, mostly just snacks, whenever she didn't feel too nauseated and her mouth wasn't hurting. She dropped ten pounds in just a few days and despaired of ever putting them back on again.

My wife's depressed appetite and unpredictable eating patterns created a problem for us. This was a side effect to chemotherapy that neither of us had anticipated.

I have mentioned a couple of dishes that I enjoyed cooking for her, like scrambled eggs with chopped chives and lightly seasoned and browned fillet of sole. What was lovingly prepared was now rudely rejected. As crazy as this sounds, as I scraped the untouched stuff off the plate into the garbage, I, too, felt rejected. When I stopped being resentful long enough to think about it, I realized that my reaction was a natural one. From feeding as primates at a prehistoric mother's breast, we humans have been conditioned to equate food with love. Throughout history, the best days have been feast days. Today, when we wish to make an evening an occasion for someone special, we take them out to dinner.

Every time I cooked up something for Chris, then had to dump it in the garbage can, it was a case, in a way, of unrequited love.

This was one of those unforeseen personal conflicts that Chris and I simply had to sit down and talk out. She told me what foods she thought might not trigger her nausea, both in preparation and on her plate.

They were mainly bland dishes, with very little cooking odor. Poached eggs. Chicken breasts simmered in milk. Salads with chopped chicken bought pre-cooked. Lightly seasoned meat loaf. And on the really bad days, or as a nourishing supplement anytime, homemade vanilla milkshakes with a little sugar, an egg, and a heaped tablespoon of malt. (The trick to making a really tasty shake is to use ice cold milk and a generous helping of frozen-hard, quality ice cream.)

I promised not to fry eggs, bacon, fish, or just about anything else without first turning on the Jenn-Air stove-top exhaust, throwing open the kitchen windows, and closing the door. In practice, I found that the best solution was just to eat what Chris ate.

She was prescribed regular vitamin and mineral supplements. These are important, both to replenish those destroyed by chemotherapy and to build up the patient's system between treatments.

A year or so later, Chris would become interested in something that up to then she had known about only vaguely. It is called alternative therapy. One aspect of it is based on the work of an American, the late Dr. Linus Pauling (Ph.D.), and others on the use of vitamins in combatting cancer. When she had read enough about it to make her own informed decision, Chris began a daily regimen of certain vitamin and mineral supplements.

"The practice is controversial," she would be quick to admit. "Dr. Pauling and his supporters have a lot of critics. I just wonder how many of them have won the Nobel Prize, as he has. Twice!"

Quite apart from the debilitating side effects of chemotherapy, Chris hated the way it affected her taste. Everything she ate or drank had a metallic taste to it. This was another reason, along with nausea and the sores that made eating unpleasant, for her food rejection. It was caused by the metal-based chemicals in the chemo she was being given.

Chris was a fastidious person. The metallic taste she could live with. The way chemotherapy made her smell, she could not.

A few days after her second chemo, she dragged herself out of bed, walked into the living-room, and plopped down on the sofa.

"I hate the word," she said, "but it's the only one for it. I stink."

She wrinkled her nose.

"I smell like a human Chernobyl."

"It's not that noticeable," I said.

"It is to me."

She had tried lashings of Shalimar perfume and cologne, layering the cologne on the perfume. It had proved to be a cosmetic band-aid. In an hour or so, Chernobyl was back.

The next week, when she was better able to get up and around, she haunted department store and Shoppers Drug Mart perfume counters. She drove heaven knows how many cosmetologists to distraction. But she finally came up with the solution. I was not surprised. In my experience with my wife, if determination was a factor, she usually did.

The answer was Youth-Dew Bath Oil by Estée Lauder, the

same cosmetics firm whose product she had found effectively concealed her facial pallor with its Self-Action Tanning Cream.

It made the bathroom smell like a rose-bed that had been run over by a steamroller, but it worked. Her pores absorbed the bath oil and retained its heavy scent.

Chris was jubilant. She practically waltzed into the living-room. Flouncing her robe as she sat down, she offered me a forearm to sniff. "Don't I smell *gorgeous?*"

She certainly did. Neither of us cared that because she had dumped so much Youth-Dew into the tub, the bathroom reeked of the stuff for hours afterward. Despite being down with Chernobyl, she had come up smelling of roses!

Just before her surgery, Chris anxiously had told Dr. Gerard McCarthy that she wanted to live to see her first grandchild. That had been two months earlier. The baby was due near the end of June. Chris not only wished to be there for this blessed event, she wanted to be well enough to enjoy it.

Over some protest that she should not interrupt her chemotherapy program of eight monthly treatments, she suspended the third one, scheduled for mid-June.

"Looking forward to that child helped me survive my surgery. she said. "I'm not about to be wrecked by chemo when I meet him. Or her. Besides, I'd be so blown away, I probably couldn't even make the drive to Calgary."

Dr. McIntyre believed, as Chris did, that willing herself to live to see her first grandchild had been a factor in keeping her alive. "I've been practising medicine for fifty years," he said. "I have found that with cancer, everything is attitude. The determination to live, for the birth of a grandchild or whatever reason, often helps to prolong life."

Chris was eagerly looking forward to something else over the next few weeks. She had been thinking about what Don McIntyre had said about "hedonism." Following her surgery for ovarian cancer, he had advised her "Get the most pleasure you can out of every new day."

On our first stay at the Leighton Artist Colony, we had taken a Banff Centre bus tour of the region. Chris fell in love with two sites the tour had visited: Moraine Lake, the looking-glass lake in the mountain frame that is pictured on our twenty-dollar bill. And Château Lake Louise.

She had been particularly enchanted with Lake Louise and the luxury resort that bears its name. History, myth, and mystique hover over the place like the low-flying clouds that sometimes get trapped by the surrounding mountains. Booking a room overlooking the lake for a week, on the penthouse floor of the Château, was my wife's choice of hedonism.

I agreed that we had a lot to celebrate. She was alive and, since she had skipped her June chemo, feeling reasonably well. Our first grandchild was scheduled to make his grand entry into the world before the end of the month. It was our thirty-seventh wedding anniversary on June 24. A week or so before that, for me, anyway, it was Father's Day. I thought it might fall a bit early for Casey.

We drove. The day after our departure, we had dinner with our son and his wife at their Calgary home. We brought gifts of a Gund "Teddy" and a lion bundle-bag for the baby. We drive into the mountains and checked into Château Lake Louise the next day.

Since some hotels and motels don't allow dogs, usually due to a bad experience with an irresponsible owner, I was concerned that Nigel might be a problem. I shouldn't have been. Château Lake Louise has style as well as substance. All three of us were checked in as registered guests, with Nigel paying $7.50 a day. A bargain rate compared to ours.

"Just look!" Chris cried out.

She was standing at the window. It was breath-taking, all right. A Van Gogh of poppies sloped down from the Château to the walkway at water's edge. The lake flawlessly mirrored glacial Mt. Victoria, named for the much-loved monarch, and the flanking mountains that kneel to her.

The management had provided a bottle of Henkell sparkling wine in a silver ice bucket. It seemed like a good time, even if it was four days early, to celebrate our anniversary. While Chris was still soaking up God's ambience, I hauled a bottle of Chambord raspberry liqueur out of my bag. I popped the bottle of German champagne and mixed a couple of kir royales.

"Here's to our thirty-seventh," I said, raising my glass.

"And to hedonism," Chris said. She flashed a smile and walked back to the window.

How good it was, after all she'd been through, to see her so happy!

Her high spirits held up.

Casey and Elaine, bearing gifts, drove up for Father's Day brunch in the Victoria Room. They returned to Calgary with Elaine promising Chris, prophetically, as it turned out, that she would "Hurry up and have the baby!"

That evening, we walked the path that separates the forest from the shoreline, down from the Château, along one side of Lake Louise. At the far end, where the path leaves the lake and begins to get rugged, rising sharply, we paused before turning back. Chris sat down on a rock.

She had seemed to be feeling generally well since leaving

Winnipeg. I was aware that sometimes, like now, this had been with some effort. She tired easily. This both frustrated and embarrassed her. It was something that she tried to conceal from everyone, even from me. Mostly, perhaps, from herself.

There was one of those gorgeous icy moons, reflected off snow-caps and glaciers, that you only get in high mountain country.

"I've seen St. Peter's in Rome," Chris mused. "Notre Dame in Paris. Westminster Abbey in London. But the Rockies are the greatest cathedral of them all." She reached out her hand to mine and pulled herself to her feet. "No contest," she grinned. "God was both the architect and the builder."

We walked along in silence, still holding hands.

"Do you believe there is a God?" I asked.

It was a dialogue that we had had before, but not since she had gotten cancer. She had told me once that she could not rationalize an all-knowing, all-seeing God who allowed so much injustice and suffering in the world He had created. I wondered if she still felt that way.

Chris didn't reply right away. "I don't know," she finally said. Then she added "It would be very comforting if I could."

The next day, we made the drive over the world-famous Icefields Parkway, from Lake Louise to Jasper. This is a three-hour drive each way, with much added time for slowdowns and stops for meandering animals, torrential rivers, spectacular waterfalls, massive glaciers, and towering mountain peaks. If you look upon the Rockies as a cathedral, as Chris said she did, or even if you don't, this drive is a spiritual experience.

When we got back, there was a message to phone Casey.

Chris made the call. She listened for a moment, then excitedly called to me across the room: "Its a boy! Born at 2:12 a.m.! Seven pounds! Both Elaine and the baby are doing just fine!"

We checked out and headed for Calgary General Hospital.

Since Casey and Elaine hadn't picked a name yet, we called our grandson "Baby Generic." It was not until two weeks or so after we got back to Winnipeg that he was dignified with the name Tyson Frederick.

Chris took two more chemo treatments. One on her return, early in July. The other about mid-August. The feelings of improved spiritual and physical well-being that she had brought home with her from Calgary and the mountains had begun to fade. She was back to Tanning Cream and Youth-Dew.

More than ever, she wanted the answers to some questions.

Does chemotherapy have a proven track record for late-stage ovarian cancer? Other than someone "going in for a little look" after eight treatments over almost as many months, how could she know if it was working?

Might no treatment be as good, perhaps even better, all things considered, than the treatment she was taking?

If she had just one year or so to live, with or without chemo, should she allow herself to be made deathly ill for most of those last few months? Where was the quality of life, whatever amount of it she had left, in that?

And finally, might chemotherapy kill not just the disease, but—in spirit, if not in fact—her too?

"I want state-of-the-art answers to those questions," Chris said matter-of-factly, "before I take one more chemo. Not just those that can be found in library books, up-to-date as they might have been when they were written. And certainly not those provided by some quick-fix question-and-answer pamphlet."

Chris was still recovering from the effects of her latest chemo treatment. She was not feeling well enough to search for the answers herself. She asked me to do it for her.

A phone call to the Canadian Cancer Society in Manitoba brought an offer of a couple of pamphlets on ovarian cancer and chemotherapy. I felt that expecting anything more than this was like trying to get a corporate decision from the branch office of a large corporation, which the Canadian Cancer Society is. The Society's head office is in Toronto.

In the United States, both the American Cancer Society and the National Cancer Institute are loosely affiliated with the Cancer Information Service, which provides Americans with a toll-free national "help line." There is no help line for Canadians. I tried the American number: 1-800-CAN-CER. I got the recorded reply, "You have dialled a number that is not available from your calling area."

Frustration followed frustration.

Chris was taking her chemotherapy at St. Boniface Hospital under the aegis of the Manitoba Cancer Treatment and Research Foundation. This organization has offices, including a large reference library, on Olivia Street in Winnipeg.

When I entered the library, there was no one there but two librarians. One was seated at a reception desk, doing paperwork. Another was checking through a bank of filing cabinets.

I told the receptionist that my wife was an ovarian cancer patient. I asked to see the latest information they had on ovarian and its treatment by chemotherapy. The woman was very agreeable. She got up, led me across the floor, and pulled a file. Before I got it open, the other librarian was at my elbow. She asked me if I was a doctor. I said no. She took the file from me, went to a phone and dialled a number. She hung up and came back.

"I'm sorry," she said, "but this library is for the use of doctors only."

I guess I should have expected something like this, but I hadn't.

"I'm sorry," the woman repeated. "Dr. Israels, our Executive Director, instructed me to ask you to leave."

I felt sandbagged. Worse still, I felt that Chris was being sandbagged. I also felt a little bitter. "When the Foundation wants money," I wondered aloud, "does it ask for the bulk of it from the doctors or the public?"

It wasn't too far down the road I got my answer. It came in the form of a plea from the Foundation that I "help conquer cancer" by making a donation of $10,000 , or more, or $25.00, or less ("all gifts are crucial"). It carried what I guessed was meant to be an impressive imprint: "From the desk of Executive Director Dr. Lyonel G. Israels, M.D." I noticed how Israels' doctorate was declared at both ends of his name, like decorative bookends.

I was not impressed.

It was just a week or so after I was turfed out of the Foundation library that I discovered Planetree. I was digging in the public library for whatever recent reports I could find on ovarian cancer and its treatment by chemotherapy when I hit paydirt.

In an article on cancer, there was mention of a personal health resource centre in San Francisco called Planetree. In general terms, it was described as a non-profit group dedicated to helping patients take an active part in their own health and medical care. Specifically, it offered to provide state-of-the-art health and medical information for a small fee.

At first, Chris and I were sceptical. There are a lot of unscrupulous groups out there, most notoriously the "miracle cure clinics," who prey on sick people. We both were aware that desperation often drives the patient with advanced cancer, and those close to them, to clutch at straws.

Its brochure dispelled any hesitation we had about Planetree. The Center has a massive back-up of medical reference books, information sources, and current literature. It is plugged into the computer databases of the U.S. Library of Medicine. Its printouts on cancer and AIDS, detailing prognosis, staging, treatment, and experimental research, are kept updated by the U.S. Cancer Institute.

What caught Chris's eye right off were the Center's founding principles.

She paraphrased the brochure.

"The name is from the planetree, or sycamore tree," Chris quoted loosely. "Hippocrates is said to have sat under one while teaching medicine in ancient Greece.

"It's symbolic. Planetree believes that many people today want to learn enough about their personal health care to be participants. They want to be able to make their own informed decisions."

Chris's expression was that of someone whose parallel view, dismissed by so many for so long, had finally been vindicated.

"Well, *hallelujah!*" she said.

The packet we got from Planetree was eight feet of computerized printout on ovarian cancer. It was the latest information of everything from Treatment Overview to Treatment by Cell Type or Stage, with Options; from Standard Treatment to Investigational; from Staging to Prognosis. It ended with a detailed list of fifteen source References.

If we still had any doubts about Planetree, they were dispelled by a doctor Chris consulted for another opinion on chemotherapy. When she took the bulky report from her purse and referred to it to ask a question, he said: "Where did you get that?" He walked around the desk, took it from her, and returned to his seat.

"For the rest of the interview," Chris said, "he just sat and read my printout. I guess my sources were more current than his sources."

Chris quit chemotherapy after the first four of her scheduled eight treatments. Her decision was based primarily on what she had learned of its probable effectiveness for someone with advanced ovarian cancer. It also was greatly influenced by her commitment to quality of life. Finally, Dr. McIntyre had advised her to do what she always tried to do: make her own informed decision.

We had gone for a walk after dinner, along the Wellington Crescent footpath, when Chris made her announcement.

"I'm not going to take any more chemo," she said.

This was no surprise to me. I had seen it coming. "If you don't believe in it . . ." I began.

She cut me off. "I never did."

We walked along in silence.

"I never felt that it was right for me," she said finally. "I always felt that despite the beliefs and best efforts of the chemotherapists, patients in my situation are time-charted wins and losses on the chemo stats sheets." She made a face. "Frankly, I always felt like a lab rat."

We came abreast of a block of tennis courts. A few people were talking, laughing, batting balls back and forth.

"I'm convinced that just putting myself in the hands of a medical team, however skilled," Chris said, "is not good enough. I feel that I have to fight this disease on all fronts. Mentally. Emotionally. With every weapon that I can muster."

In her continuing research on cancer, she had read estimates that one in four patients in the United Kingdom, one in five in Canada and the United States, complement conventional medicine with some other form of treatment.

"There's a whole arsenal of weapons out there that I haven't even looked at," she said.

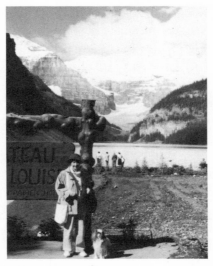

Château Lake Louise. Summer '87 — "I've seen St. Peter's in Rome. Notre Dame in Paris. Westminster Abbey in London. But the Rockies are the greatest cathedral of them all," Chris said. "God was both the architect and the builder."

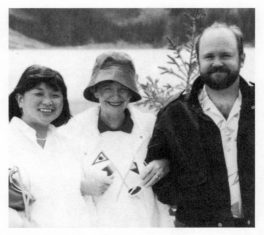

With Casey and Elaine. Lake Louise. Summer '87 — Casey and Elaine, bearing gifts, drove up for Father's Day brunch in the Victoria Room. They returned to Calgary with Elaine promising Chris, prophetically, as it turned out, that she would "Hurry up and have the baby!"

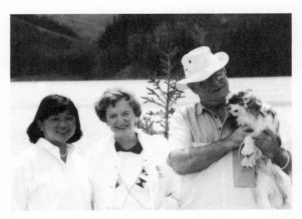

With Elaine, Nigel, and me. Lake Louise. Summer '87 — She had been particularly enchanted with Lake Louise and the luxury resort that bears its name. History, myth, and mystique hover over the place like the low-flying clouds that sometimes get trapped by the surrounding mountains.

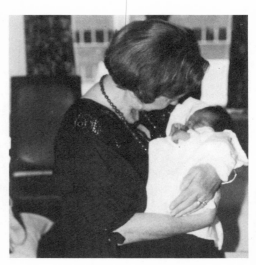

Calgary General Hospital. Summer '87 — Dr. McCarthy told Chris he thought she had a 30 percent chance of survival. "I told him that I was expecting my first grandchild in June," Chris said. "That I had to live at least until then."

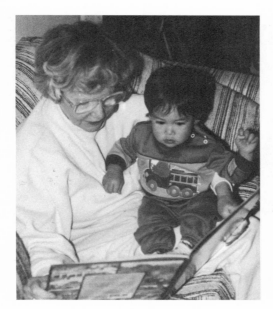

With grandson Tyson. Calgary. Fall '88 — Dr. McIntyre believed that willing herself to live to see her first grandchild had been a factor in keeping Chris alive. "The determination to live often helps to prolong life."

6 · Visuals, vitamins, and apricot pits

If the world of cancer and conventional cancer treatment is shadowy, the world of alternative treatment is even more so. It is dismissed as foolishness, or quackery, or ridiculed as "black magic" by the majority of medical professionals.

Why then, Chris wondered, are increasing numbers of sick people, including cancer patients, turning to it to complement conventional treatment? A few days earlier, she had described alternative treatment as "an arsenal that she hadn't even looked at" in her personal war on cancer.

"What I have to try to find out," said Chris, "is whether it's an arsenal of blanks or live ammunition."

Do alternative therapies work? Do some work and not others? Or are they just a desperate alternative for the seriously ill, when conventional treatment has not produced hoped-for results?

Chris soon learned that getting the answers to these questions is much more difficult than it sounds. There are no hard-and-fast studies on what works and what doesn't in alternative treatment.

There is no proof anything does.

It is primarily a world of faith and, unless the experience is personal, generally hearsay successes.

After about a month of chasing down reference library sources on the subject, Chris came up with a pretty comprehensive overview. She read to me from her notes.

"I've found seven major alternative therapies: Acupuncture. Visualization. Vitamins. Touch. Diet. Laetrile. And Spiritual.

"Diet is the least controversial. Laetrile the most."

Laetrile works on the same principle as chemotherapy. The drug laetrile, which contains cyanide, is extracted from apricot pits. It is injected into the patient. As in chemo, the intent is to poison the cancerous cells to retard, shrink, or eliminate the tumor. Most sources of laetrile and clinics that administer the drug are in Mexico.

"Like all alternative therapies," said Chris, "laetrile has its supporters and its detractors. Many cancer patients swear by it and claim 'cures.' Just as many others have showed no change. Still others have died when they chose laetrile over conventional treatment."

In this game of life and death choices into which she had been thrust, my wife tried to calculate the odds and, whenever possible, hedge her bets. How to handle alternative therapy was one of those choices.

"I am considering some types of alternative therapy as a complement to conventional medical treatment," she said. "I would never adopt them as an outright substitute."

Many critics of alternative therapies argue that their so-called "successes" are a result of the "placebo effect."

In clinical trials, half a group of patients are given the actual medicine to be tested. The other half are given placebos that just appear to be the same. Patients known to their doctors to be hypochondriacs, suffering from imagined illnesses, sometimes are given placebos.

"Almost invariably," said Chris, "they feel much relief, or make remarkable recoveries, from whatever it is that doesn't ail them."

This argument, made by detractors of alternative therapies, holds that they, too, can accomplish nothing in themselves. That they are, in effect, placebos that work only because the patient believes they will.

Chris had a candid response to this.

"I really don't care whether they work because they work, or only because I believe they work," she said. "Just as long as they work!"

The least controversial of the alternatives are the various diet and detoxification therapies. They originated in Austria in the early 1900s and are said to have a track record of improved survival rates.

"These diets are based on organic fruits and vegetables," Chris said, "together with the elimination of refined, processed, salted foods and fats. The patient also is given certain vitamins and minerals. An important aspect of the treatment is detoxification, or the ridding of the body of poisonous wastes.

"It's fascinating to me that while some therapies, like chemo and laetrile, dose the patient with poison, others, like the diet ones, strive to eliminate them."

It also struck her as significant that there is growing emphasis on diet as a factor in cancer prevention. "No one denies that what we eat can have an effect on whether or not we are made more susceptible to some forms of cancer," she said. "This includes the medical profession. It is even thought by some medical researchers and practitioners that the only real 'cure' for cancer is in its prevention, to a great degree through diet. The controversy lies in whether diet can have a positive effect on someone who already has cancer."

Two alternative therapies that caught Chris's interest were Linus Pauling's Vitamin C and Carl Simonton's Visualization.

Pauling, who died at 93 in Big Sur, California, in 1994, twice won the Nobel Prize. One award was for his campaign against nuclear weapons. The other was in the field of chemistry. Dr. Pauling contended that daily megadoses of Vitamin C would act both to prevent cancer and to extend the lifespan of cancer patients.

"His theories are controversial," Chris said. "Like so many in alternative therapy, one study supports them. Another doesn't. One argument put forward by proponents is that the negative studies are stacked: Cancer patients usually have reached an advanced stage before turning to alternative therapies.

"Pauling also claims that these studies involve patients whose immune systems already have been damaged by chemotherapy. Those who believe in vitamins and minerals as alternative therapies argue that this could inhibit, or even negate, their effectiveness."

Chris had a characteristic reaction to detractors of megadose Vitamin C therapy: "Who am I to argue with Linus Pauling? Besides," she added philosophically, "taking all that Vitamin C may or may not have an effect on my cancer, but I'll probably never get another cold!"

She began by taking 10,000 milligrams of Vitamin C daily. Eventually, as she learned more about vitamin and mineral therapy, she added Vitamins A and B-complex, E, Beta-carotene, and the minerals Selenium and Potassium.

"Vitamin C plays a known role in strengthening the immune system," Chris said. "A deficiency lowers the number of specialized white blood cells called T-cells, that defend us against disease."

Vitamin C also counters the action of chemicals used commercially to preserve meat. Without Vitamin C, these additives, called nitrates and nitrites, are known to increase the threat of cancer.

Chris's research came up with Vitamin A and Beta-carotene, which the body converts into Vitamin A, and Vitamins B-complex and E as "thought to have a preventive—even a combative—effect on some forms of cancer."

She found the same optimistic reports of diets supplemented with Potassium and Selenium.

"In trials over lengthy periods, in clinics from the United States to Germany, Japan to Italy," said Chris, "researchers are reporting positive results from these vitamins and minerals. They're not claiming 'cures,' but they are suggesting longer life expectancy."

In all of these studies, a complementary, or compatible diet is recommended: fruits and vegetables daily, with emphasis on those high in natural sources of Vitamin C and Beta-carotene. We began eating a lot of apples, oranges, grapefruit, apricots, carrots, cabbage, Brussels sprouts, spinach, beet tops and beets, and sweet potatoes. "Generally speaking," said Chris, "the darker green the vegetable, the more nutritious it is."

We also began breakfasting on old-fashioned oatmeal with raisins and increasing our fibre intake with peas, various kinds of beans, and parsnips. Potatoes always had been a staple, but now they came baked, with skins also eaten. Never as French fries. Nothing, as a matter of fact, was deep-fried. We ate far less meat—smaller servings with the fat cut off. Finally, and the toughest cut of all, we threw our salt shakers away.

It was not hard for me to adapt my eating habits to Chris's. Without frying, salting, and smothering your food in fatty sauces and gravies, you begin to get the actual, subtle flavors of whatever it is that you're eating. I found this, in particular, with fresh vegetables. After a while, imagined or not, you begin to hear your body shouting "Hurrah!"

Dr. Carl Simonton is an American radiation oncologist. Chris adopted his visualization technique as her other alternative therapy because it is rooted in the power of the mind. She always had believed that if negative thinking could add to your degree of illness, which hardly anyone disputes, positive thinking logically could have an equal and opposite effect: It could contribute to wellness.

"This is the basis for the Simonton and similar techniques of visualization, or mind's eye, therapy," said Chris. "Basically, it means thinking positively. Picturing your healthy cells as heroic warriors and your sick ones as craven cowards. It means seeing your inner self as a battlefield, with the disciplined, heroic cells warring against the confused, cowardly ones.

"And winning. Always winning.

"It means seeing beauty and peace within yourself, where you have been told there is only ugly and disruptive disease. In a phrase," she summarized, "it is the ultimate triumph of mind over matter."

Visualization can be considered the humanist side of spiritual therapy. The difference between them is that visualization is rooted in the concept of the body healing itself, on command from the patient's own mind, or spirit. Spiritual therapy is based on the patient asking for help from a Higher Power.

"I would never question that 'more things are wrought by prayer than this world dreams of,'" said Chris. "I also am prepared to accept documented evidence, in records kept by mainstream religions, of 'faith healing.' But I have no time for the tent and television evangelists who prey on the desperately ill and sell 'miracle cures' like used cars."

Acupuncture and Therapeutic Touch, or "TT," were the other two alternative therapies that Chris researched. Acupuncture has been practised in China for a few thousand years. It is based on the principle of a "Life Force," which has been shared by all societies, in one form or another, since the beginning of recorded time.

The Chinese believe that twelve lines of this force course through the body, one to each vital organ, and that they can be influenced by the insertion of pins. Surgery as intolerably painful as for cancer of the brain has been carried out in China without anaesthetic. It was done with the strategic insertion of four pins, while the patient remained conscious.

Because she considered it primarily an alternative therapy for pain control, which was not now a problem with her, Chris did not try acupuncture. She did, however, get involved in therapeutic touch. With her remarkable capacity for finding out things (*Sometimes I thought, "Lord only knows how!"*) she came up with the name of a woman practitioner who holds sessions in Winnipeg's west end.

"'TT'" Chris explained to me, "is another therapy based on 'Life Force.' It has nothing to do with the 'laying on of hands,' or 'faith healing,' both of which have been so commercialized on television. The practitioner's hands never actually touch the subject.

"We discussed my illness and surgeries," Chris said. "Then the woman simply concentrated and passed her hands slowly over the lower part of my body, where I had had the colon and ovarian tumors. She did this in silence for about fifteen minutes. I felt relaxed. I experienced a sort of physical inner peace."

Chris could see that I looked a little sceptical. I spent a lot of years as a hard-nosed newspaperman on major dailies across Canada. When someone saws someone in half, I want to see the blood.

"I was sceptical, too," said Chris. "She told me to hold the palms of my hands about a half-inch apart. To concentrate on them. Then to slowly pass them back and forth. 'You will feel the Life Force,' she said."

My wife did.

When I tried it, so did I.

I was reminded of an interview I had done years earlier when I was a young reporter on *The Vancouver Province*. My subject was a postgraduate psychology student who had just returned from a year's study of yoga, in India. He was doing his best to explain to me how by disciplining the mind, as well as the body, we can reach a potential that most of us would never dream possible.

I must have looked sceptical then, too.

He stopped talking and we sat for a few moments in silence. Then he pointed to an old oak grandfather's clock that occupied a corner of the living-room. "Listen," he said.

For the first time, I heard its pendulous "tick-tock! tick-tock!"

"A small case-in-point," he said. "Because you were concentrating on your interview, your mind let you hear only what you wanted to hear. Disciplining your mind to be that selective, on command, is the next step." He smiled a little ruefully, as though he himself were still learning to crawl, before he could walk. "It's a big one," he said.

When I told my wife this story, she said that it may be an even bigger step to get the majority of doctors to abandon what she described as "MV," or "microscope vision."

"It's like tunnel vision," said Chris, "only it's done through a microscope. The doctor with MV only sees what can be mounted on a glass slide. His only reality is physical."

Frequently in her research, Chris had come across the statement that medicine in the Western World is unsurpassed in its treatment of physical trauma. Conversely, it is often described as having failed miserably in treating chronic illness.

"If a patient's condition can't be fixed with a scalpel, a splint, or a pill," Chris said, "the doctor with MV not only can't handle it, he doesn't believe it actually exists."

The opposite to this is the practice of homeopathic, or holistic medicine. "As the name suggests," said Chris, "it means the treating of 'the whole person,' spiritual as well as physical, not just that part of the patient that is diseased.

"It was what Hippocrates taught, twenty-three centuries ago in ancient Greece, when he said that it is just as important to know the patient as the disease the patient has."

Chris had read that Prince Charles, his mother the Queen, and the Queen Mother, all have homeopathic doctors. So has former U.S. President Ronald Reagan and his wife Nancy.

"When you think of the access that princes, queens, and presidents have to the best medical care in the world," she said, "you have to ask yourself: What do they know that I don't?"

Charles pinpointed the answer in an address to members

of the British Medical Association at the gala celebration of its 150th anniversary. Some of the gala went out of the occasion when he said that one of the association's "least attractive traits" is its "deeply ingrained suspicion and downright hostility towards anything unorthodox or unconventional."

"The doctors went further into shock," Chris said, "when Charles went on to champion alternative therapies as complementary to conventional medicine. He then described as 'frightening' the way drugs are prescribed as 'the universal panacea for our ills.'

"'Wonderful as some of them may be,'" he added, "'doctors should stress that health is most often determined by diet, behavior, and environment.'

"When Charles's address was reported the next day in the British press," Chris said, "there was a groundswell of reaction. The British public wanted to know more. The British Medical Association had little choice but to set up an enquiry into alternative therapies.

"The report was made public last year," Chris said. "It could find no scientific proof that treatment by any of the alternative therapies works.

"The charitable way to describe that report," she said, "is to echo its own operative word: 'scientific.' The polite way is to describe it as predictable. The realistic way is to call it a whitewash of conventional medical thinking in most of the Western World."

Chris found a few promising straws of change in the wind.

"Early on, when I asked a consulting doctor about visualization," Chris said, "he smiled benignly at me—like I was the village idiot." A couple of years later, when she dropped in for another consultation, she noticed pamphlets on the Simonton technique displayed at the reception desk in his office.

"Some of the more progressive clinics and hospitals," she said, "are beginning to look long and hard at alternative therapies. Pain centres are studying acupuncture and touch therapy. Cancer patients are being offered visualization counselling.

"We seem to be moving, however slowly, towards the holistic healing that our ancestors practised many centuries ago," said Chris, "and that we somehow lost sight of along the way."

Even before she began her ongoing research on cancer, Chris had always brought home armloads of books from the library. She had always wanted to know as much as she could about just about everything.

Three years earlier, when she had undergone colon surgery, we had been dismayed by our ignorance of the appalling disease that had invaded our lives. The books then had been about cancer and the conventional medical procedures used in treating it. Over the past year or so, most of the books that Chris brought home had been about alternative therapies.

Comfortably curled up in the sofa-chair in the living-room, with Nigel sandwiched in beside her, she liked to read them in the evening. When she came across a passage that she thought was particularly interesting, she read it out loud. She did a lot of this reading aloud for my benefit. On this particular evening, she was reading about Dr. Bernard Siegel, a New Haven, Connecticut, surgeon.

"This is a very interesting guy," said Chris. "A visualization workshop he attended, given by Carl Simonton, inspired him to make his practice as spiritual and psychological as it was surgical. For starters, he dropped the 'Dr. Siegel' and became just 'Bernie' to his patients.

"He moved his desk off to one side so that they sat and spoke on equal terms. Instead of seeing himself as a healer, he recast himself in the role of trying to help patients live long enough to heal themselves."

Never mind that I was watching Monday Night Football on television and it was probably fourth down and goal to go. What my wife was telling me got my attention.

This was because Bernie Siegel had some startling stuff to say. In a survey of his cancer patients, he discovered that only about one in five was willing to dedicate themselves to staying alive.

"The rest," Chris paraphrased Bernie, "were divided. Most refused to stop self-destructing by quitting smoking, adopting a new diet, or changing lifestyles. The rest wanted to die. They saw what they perceived as their imminent death from cancer as a release from problems they couldn't face. Or as a punishment to themselves or others.

"He says the fighters are generally looked upon as 'bad patients.'"

Without being conscious that she was doing it, Chris switched to the personal pronoun. "We want to know what tests, treatment, and drugs are being given us, and why. When a doctor tells us we have this or that much time left, we're inclined to ask ourselves: *What does he know? He may be a good doctor, but he's not God!*

"Bernie doesn't look upon us as the 'bad patients'" said Chris. "He calls us the 'exceptional ones.'"

I couldn't help grinning. There were a couple of doctors who I figured looked upon Chris, by Bernie's definition, as pretty "exceptional!"

As well as diet and lifestyle, his self-help formula for cancer patients concentrates on getting rid of stress, resolving conflicts, and creating positive self-images.

Chris quoted him on alternative therapies: "'It's absurd not to use treatments that work, just because we don't yet understand them.'

"He holds that 'unconditional love is the most powerful stimulant to the immune system,'" said Chris. "He writes: 'If I told patients to raise their blood levels of immune globulins, or T-cells, no one would know how, but if I can teach them to love themselves and others fully, the same changes happen automatically. The truth is, love heals.'

"Bernie encourages patients to have faith in God, too," Chris concluded, "but in the context of 'God helps those who help themselves.' He suggests that we shouldn't expect Him to do all the work!"

Chris's own combination of conventional medicine and alternative therapies was working for her. Going into fall and winter, after her surgery for ovarian cancer in the spring and the chemotherapy she quit in late summer, she felt great and she looked great.

She was determinedly practising the alternative therapies of vitamins, diet, and visualization. I was her active partner in the last two, but not the first. I believe that a normally healthy person who eats properly, and is not under unusual physical stress, does not need vitamin supplements. The exception I made, after reading Chris's notes on vitamins as an alternative therapy, was Vitamin C. As a boost to my immune system, particularly against colds, I began a normal dose of 250 milligrams daily.

On line with Linus Pauling's program for cancer patients, Chris was taking a megadose of forty times that much.

At first, without realizing it, we had cheated on visualization. We had attempted it when we had nothing better to do, or when we had fallen into bed, half asleep, after "The Late Show."

"This isn't working," Chris said. "All I can picture is something from the fridge and a good night's sleep."

I agreed. When you've been married to someone long enough, you sometimes experience a sort of mental telepathy. I had been "visualizing" a plate of cheese and crackers and a cold glass of milk.

We both began to realize that visualization is something you have to work at. I referred back to the postgraduate student I had met in Vancouver. Chris and I decided that while you don't have to be an expert in yoga to be successful at visualization, you do have to be capable of closing your mind to outside distractions. Like the "tick-tock" of a clock. You also have to shut out distractions from within. Like thoughts of a bedtime snack.

I knew Chris had been both disappointed and a little discouraged by our first week of failed attempts. She rallied us both now with the suggestion that we take a whole new approach.

"What do you say?" she prompted.

As if I had a choice!

She set up a schedule of two sessions daily: first thing in the morning, when she was well rested, and early in the evening, before she began getting tired. We had one of those bedside digital clocks with a buzz alarm. Each session, which took place at about the same time every morning and evening, was timed for twenty minutes. Because soft music is a mood-setter, Chris decided to find something appropriate for background for our sessions.

"It has to be instrumental," she said. "Vocals would be a distraction."

Nothing in our modest library of recorded music struck Chris as the right stuff. Like most teen-age girls from the forties, she had been a Frank Sinatra fan ever since his debut as a bow-tied anorexic, swoon-crooning with the Tommy Dorsey orchestra. A lovesick Old Blue Eyes singing "set 'em up Joe" certainly set a mood. But I had to agree it was the wrong mood, and anyway, vocals were out.

I was shuffling through our cassettes of instrumental music when I came across Wagner. I held it up for Chris to see.

"How about 'Ride of the Valkyries?'" I asked, straight-faced.

I ducked the sofa pillow she threw at me.

A couple of years earlier, we had seen Robert Redford and Meryl Streep in *Out of Africa*. I remembered how much we had enjoyed both the movie and the soundtrack. I checked with a music shop in Polo Park Mall and was told it was available on cassette from MCA records. I ordered one.

It is played by the Academy of St. Martin-in-The-Fields, with Neville Marriner conducting. The music on Side A is wonderfully relaxing. At times it is haunting, even mystical. Especially when an African choir sings the traditional "Siyawe." I suppose you could call this a vocal, but it doesn't sound like one. The combined voices come off like a richly melodious musical instrument.

When the cassette came in and I auditioned it for Chris, she thought it was just right. Coincidentally, Side A ran almost exactly twenty minutes, the length of time that she had set for each session. We tried it that same evening.

When you do visualization at home without benefit of a leader, as you have in visualization workshops, you have to find what works for you. The mood set by the music, and her own interpretation of the visualization technique, worked for Chris.

I asked her, after that first evening session was over, how she had handled it.

At the start of films and videotapes, there is a ten-second visual countdown: a circle around a "10"—"9"—"8" down to "0," with each number "wiped" in turn, as though by a sweep-second hand.

"When the music started," said Chris, "I closed my eyes and pictured that countdown. I wanted to focus in on myself as fully as I could, and to begin the images that I would see with my mind's eye."

The images began within herself. She described it as a sort of Cook's tour of her body, seeking out the places where the cancer had been found. Along the way she repeated over and over again, "I have the ability to heal myself."

"I *can* heal myself! I *will* heal myself!"

She pictured the T-cells of her immune system as the cells in the white hats. The cancer cells were those in the black hats. "At each encounter," she said, "it was just like always: The guys in the white hats hammered the guys in the black hats!"

With the good cells in command, her mind's-eye tour then took her back to her childhood.

"When I was a teenager, spending my summers at 'Ramona,'" Chris said, "I liked to paddle off by myself to some of the fourteen thousand islands on Lake of the Woods. Some, near our own island cottage, were too small for more than a small patch of grass, and maybe a tree or two. I would beach my canoe and lie in the grass, looking up at the sky."

She told me how she would pass a languid hour or two dreaming a young girl's dreams. Or working the white clay of the clouds into fanciful sculptures.

"I can visualize myself as that young girl again. My body is strong and healthy. I have so very much to live for. I try to feel the warmth, as I did then, of a summer that I don't believe will ever end."

My own visualization was much different. I concentrated on trying to project some of my wellness to the woman who lay on the bed opposite mine. I pictured myself as a transmitter, sending a message of health. It did not surprise Chris when she asked me what I had visualized and I told her. She knew I believed that we are all connected, in some way that we don't yet understand, to the "Life Force" that created and governs the universe.

Chris once explained to a friend, a little irreverently I thought: "Fred thinks each one of us is a little Pop from The Big Bang."

Chris never allowed herself to become preoccupied with cancer, but she never tried to pretend that she didn't have it, either, "I feel good now," she'd say from out-of-the-blue, "but I have a chronic disease. I always have to remember that."

To reinforce her determination to fight diseased cells, she made a fist whenever she thought of them. Throughout the day, she practised reaffirmation. Sometimes just to herself. Sometimes out loud, as though to reassure both of us that she would never give up the good fight.

"I belong to a special group," she would say. "We are doing something about our disease that others don't. The statistics don't apply to us."

She was referring to predicted life expectancies based on

staging of the various cancers. A few months earlier, Chris had been told that it was unlikely she would live to see another Christmas. She didn't believe a word of it.

"As well as my own positive attitude," she said, "what will help keep me alive is Don McIntyre's hedonism."

The "Hedonism Principle" is simple: You must always be doing something that gives you pleasure, or looking forward to something that will. Since we both very much enjoyed live concert music, we bought two season tickets to the Winnipeg Symphony's masterworks series, presented from fall into late spring.

The doctor who had predicted my wife's death within months was a new one she had approached for an opinion. He had based it on her planned substitution of alternative therapy for chemotherapy. I was furious and told him so. I thought it was mindlessly cruel of him to make so negative a statement to someone who was trying so hard to be positive.

It didn't bother Chris as much as it did me.

Reading books by doctor-converts like Bernie Siegel and Carl Simonton had prepared her for this sort of professional myopia. When we picked up our season tickets to the concerts, she joked about it. "If I'm not around after Christmas," she said, "you'll be stuck with an empty seat."

I was still doing a slow burn over what she called the "Doomsday Prophesy," but I had to grin. "I'll take that chance," I said.

We had stopped going to dog shows because her cancer had made it impossible for Chris actively to take part in them. As a result, we had lost contact with a lot of "dog people" we had enjoyed meeting and competing with over the years. Chris decided now that this had been a mistake.

She got reflective one fall evening while we were out walking Nigel. "We always enjoyed watching all the breeds compete for points in conformation and obedience," she said. "Not just Ms. Liz and Beau and the rest of the Standard Poodles. It's a mistake to lose that, just because of this damned disease!"

It was yet another reaffirmation of her promise, both to herself and to me, that she would not give in to it.

"I can't let cancer take charge of any part of my life," she said.

The first week in December, we attended three days of shows sponsored by the Northwinds Dog Club. They were the first we had been to since Chris's cancer had decided us to stop showing. We were looking forward to Northwinds. Chris and I had always considered these among the best of the dozen or so weekends of shows that are held regionally through the year.

Although Chris was born in Winnipeg, and I spent some years there, neither of us ever understood why so many Winnipeggers take such a perverse delight in their miserably cold winters. These people brag that someone once asked Queen Elizabeth, after a Royal Visit, what was the coldest place in Canada. She replied instantly: "The corner of Portage and Main in downtown Winnipeg!"

Northwinds subscribes to this peculiar Winnipeg pride. Its emblem is of a snow-white Jack Frost, cheeks puffed, blowing a cloud of ice crystals. The motif is Christmas. The great Convention Centre hall is costumed in bright reds and greens. Poinsettias give a merry look to the judges' and officials' tables. Over the din of dogs, groomers, spectators, and the PA system calling handlers to one of the three show rings, you can almost hear the sound of sleighbells.

Chris and I enjoyed speaking with a lot of old friends.

Many of them had heard that she had cancer and expressed their concern, some a little more self-consciously than others. That awkwardness didn't bother Chris anymore. "I've had a lot of practice living with this disease, talking about it," she said later. "Most people haven't.

"What do you say to someone with cancer?" she wondered aloud. Before I could offer any suggestions, she provided a few of her own.

"'I'm glad it's you instead of me!' which is a perfectly human reaction.

"'I'm so sorry!' which sounds like the pity the cancer patient doesn't want.

"'What a rotten break!'" she concluded, "which is my personal choice."

We thoroughly enjoyed watching the dozens of breeds in conformation, second-guessing the judges with our own selections. We ached a little for the owners in the obedience ring whose dogs just yawned, got up, and walked off. We came to our feet, with the rest of the spectators, during the always exciting, sometimes hilarious, scent hurdle races.

On the drive home, after judging of the Best in Show on the final evening, I asked Chris if she were glad we'd gone.

"Absolutely!" she said.

I thought the weekend of shows might have been a little much. Like most of the "dog people" we knew, Chris and I always had come away happy but tired at the end of the three days. Walking around on a cement floor from early morning to evening, meeting and talking with people, the noise, the excitement—"It all makes for a long weekend," I said.

Chris shrugged at that. "I never should have let my cancer keep us from something we enjoy so much."

The candlelight service at First Presbyterian, our three Christmas trees, Christmas itself, all came and went with the "Doomsday Prophesy" unfulfilled. Because of her roots, hogmanay, the Scottish New Year, had been important over the years to Chris and her family.

Well, maybe not as much to Chris as to her Scottish-born parents. She wasn't too enthusiastic about haggis, although we did have it on one completely forgettable occasion. And hogmanay was, after all, just one day, however traditionally important in her heritage. I could see that Chris was looking around for something to look forward to.

The masterworks concert series had been hedonism of the classical music kind. The Northwinds Dog Shows had been the canine show kind. Chris next seized upon the world-class sports kind. The XV Olympic Winter Games were set for sixteen days in Calgary, beginning on Saturday, February 13. We had not seen our grandson, Tyson, since his birth the previous June. We had left Calgary with an open invitation from Casey and Elaine to "come back soon!" We phoned to say we'd be arriving on Friday, February 12.

"Your dad and I are coming to see the Winter Olympics," Chris told Casey, "as well as our world-class grandson!"

We left Winnipeg by car on Thursday. It was 30 degrees below Fahrenheit. No doubt it was much colder than that at the corner of Portage and Main. I don't know what the wind-chill factor was. I didn't *want* to know.

Winter driving is an adventure in the Midwest. Anyone with any sense carries a survival kit in the trunk of their car. Ours consisted of a five-gallon jerry can of gasoline. An arctic-class sleeping-bag. A hatchet. A couple of flares. A powerful lantern with spare battery. A can of Sterno. A capped jar stuffed with wood matches. A box of chocolate bars and soup-mix powders. A saucepan, soup-spoon, and a couple of mugs. A mickey of brandy. And a box of candles.

On cold winter nights in Winnipeg, guests at house parties dash out into the street every hour or so to start up and rev their cars. This is to make sure they'll start when it's time to go home. Chris and I heard it discussed at many of these parties whether one lighted candle in a car will keep you from freezing to death. I never heard the question resolved to everyone's satisfaction. So a box of candles went into our survival kit. I just hoped that we never had to get the definitive answer the hard way.

About fifty miles east of Regina, on the Trans-Canada Highway, we ran into a white-out. A white-out occurs in a heavy blizzard when the wind-blown snow is slanting into your windshield, and you can't see to drive.

You have to experience one to believe it. Having done a lot of winter driving in various parts of Canada, I had run into some pretty heavy snowstorms. I never had seen a full-blown white-out until I moved to the Midwest. If it continues long enough, snow piles up and chokes the roads. You find yourself sitting in a stranded car, whipped by a wind-chill in the minus-forties or worse, hoping you won't run out of gas before the ploughs get through.

Sometimes it takes them until the next day. That's when you're glad you've got a survival kit in the trunk of your car.

The white-out Chris, Nigel, and I drove into was rapidly moving east, while I could still see well enough to keep cautiously creeping west. After about half-an-hour, we left it behind. When we pulled into the Journey's End Motel, in Swift Current, we heard that fields by the highway were littered with cars caught up in the brunt of the storm. Fortunately, the falling and blowing snow hadn't set up any serious roadblocks. We were told that ploughs, followed by tow trucks, had been able to get through to the cars and their occupants within a couple of hours.

The visit with Casey, Elaine, and our grandson was great for both of us, but especially so for Chris. Casey, who now worked in economic development for the City of Calgary, managed to get us ringside seats for the opening ceremonies of the Olympics. When we got back to the house, we were still enthusing over the sweep, the color, the sheer spectacle of it all. Chris put it best by putting it simply. She said to Casey and Elaine: "Calgary did itself proud today."

Over the next week, Chris had to sandwich her private visualization times between the daily activities they had planned for us. Days were for Olympic pin-trading, shopping, sightseeing, and visiting "must-see" places like the Glenbow Museum. Nights were for playing with Tyson and catching the day's Olympic action on television, usually over a bowl of Häagen-Dazs ice cream.

Two of those evenings were particularly special.

Chris and I had met Mary Osaka, Elaine's mother, when Tyson was born. Soft-spoken and gracious, she was visiting with a son from her home in Raymond, Alberta. We took Casey, Elaine, and Mary to the Sheaf of Wheat dining-room, in the Skyline Hotel, for dinner. Later, we all went to Casey's office for a "box seat" to the day's medals presentation. Just below, thirty thousand people, most of them holding lighted "Olympic torches," crowded Olympic Square. A floor show came after the presentation of the medals, followed by a spectacular laser light show and fireworks display.

The other very special evening was an "Olympics Night" that Chris and I spent with Casey and Elaine at Calgary's Austrian Club. It was an invitational affair, with an impressive guest list: The Lieutenant-Governor of Alberta. The Austrian Ambassador to Canada, from Ottawa. The RCMP Commissioner for Alberta. The Austrian member of the International Olympics Committee.

Miss World, who was Austrian, also was present, along with an oom-pah-pah band and a quartet of yodelers, all wearing alpine hats and leather pants. Chris and I were chatting with the Olympic representative from Austria when a young hostess came to our table and asked to take our orders. She returned shortly with drinks and hors d'oeuvres, then went on to another table. The Olympic representative asked "Do you know who that is?"

He smiled a little when Chris and I looked mystified.

"That's Beatrix Schuba," he said. "The Austrian 1972 Olympic and World figure skating champion."

Apparently she was in Calgary to act as a public relations hostess for the Austrian Olympic Committee.

Chris said later that I just about fell off my chair. So did she. Chris studied both ballet and figure skating as a youngster in Winnipeg. I have been a figure skating fan since I was a teenager in Ottawa.

A few of us used to go down to the Minto Club and watch Barbara Ann Scott—"B.A." to us and the rest of her young friends—practising school figures and free-skate routines. It was just a few years later, in 1947 and 1948, that she became first World, then Olympic Champion.

Chris and I managed to get into a fairly lengthy conversation with Beatrix Schuba on her next trip to our table. Beatrix favored East Germany's Katarina Witt to win the women's gold, which she did. We had picked Katarina too, but our sentimental favorites were Canadian Elizabeth Manley, who gave the performance of her career to pull off the silver, and Japan's supercharged contender, Midori Ito.

The Japanese skater, who "came on like gang-busters!" as Chris put it, was a crowd but not a judge-pleaser. She finished fifth.

Some of the Olympic spirit must have rubbed off on Chris. When we got back to Winnipeg, she was more determined than ever to win the gold in her competition with cancer. She had kept up her program of megadose vitamins while we were in Calgary. She had watched carefully what she ate and drank. She had privately practised visualization at quiet times during the day. Now that we were back home, she resumed her structured sessions twice daily to the music from *Out of Africa*.

In all the hundreds of interviews with coaches and athletes that had been televised during the sixteen days of the Games, one had stuck out in Chris's mind.

"It was with a sports psychologist with one of the European ski teams," she said. "He was explaining why most teams now are being 'coached' by psychologists, as well as actual coaches."

Leading up to a previous summer Olympics, a coach and a sports psychologist conducted an experiment. Each of three basketball teams was prepared in a different way. One team was given the usual floor practice. The second was given no floor practice, but extensive "win" counselling. The third was given both.

"The teams were tested for overall improvement," Chris said. "The two that got either floor practice or psychological counselling were about equal. The team that came out on top was the one that had been given both."

Based on this, Chris decided to try to get back into the

"jalking" she had done before her surgery for ovarian cancer. She had read, too, that regular exercise is an important way to reduce the chance of getting breast cancer, or to help fight its return if you already have it. Finally, she knew that exercise was good for the mind, "which makes it doubly good for the body."

In late March, when spring began its comeback in Winnipeg, Chris and I resumed our morning "jalks," an unstressful combination of jogging and walking, along the footpath on Wellington Crescent.

7·Three strikes (but not out!)

Chris and I had no idea, when we were having so much fun at the Olympics in February, that we would be back in Calgary in October. This time, though, it would not be any fun.

Four years had passed since a chronic bowel obstruction had put Chris in hospital for surgery for colon cancer. One year ago, another tumor and an effusion of ascites had resulted in her hospitalization for surgery for ovarian cancer. Symptoms of both cancers returned in September.

As usual, her ovarian cancer, the "silent killer," approached in silence: There was no real warning of its renewed presence until Chris's stomach again began to swell.

It was in the middle of the night that I woke to see her standing by my bed. One hand was pressed against the lower part of her body. The other was gently pushing my shoulder.

When you live with someone who has cancer, your mindset, even in sleep, is always at the ready, like a smoke alarm. I came instantly and fully awake and clasped the hand on my shoulder. "What is it?"

Some nights when Chris was hurting, or she was having

deep downs about having cancer, what Ernest Hemingway used to call "black ass days," she would wake me up like this. She would sit on the edge of the bed and tell me that she was having sharp, stabbing pains. Or she would just bow her head a little and say something like "Oh, God, Fred, I'm so scared!"

Without being able to see her eyes in the darkness, I knew they were beseeching me to do something. At times like this, I would take her in my arms and hold her. We both knew that that was all I could do. For her, it was enough.

On this night, Chris was not just hurting, or depressed.

"I have to go to the hospital," she said.

I knew that Chris had been having bowel obstruction and considerable pain in her lower body for several days. Sometimes when this happened, it just went away. This time it hadn't. We got dressed. I got the "happy bag." We drove to The Misery. Chris was admitted to Emergency.

She was hurting. She was scared. She was foolishly embarrassed that she had had to haul me out of bed in the middle of the night. But she still had her sense of humor.

Parked again in the corridors of sick, injured, and wounded who make up "gurney row," she was examined by the duty doctor. He asked a few questions and pushed and probed a little. He told her that she was going to be admitted.

Chris grinned at me. "I wonder whose territory it is this time?" Under the circumstances, it was a pretty funny line. Morris Broder had done her colon surgery. Gerard McCarthy her ovarian. "I guess until they run some tests," she said, her grin broadening, "I'm up for grabs."

The tests began the next day. A barium enema and X-ray showed a narrowing of the sigmoid colon. Digital pelvic examinations disclosed that this was because of a large tumor that was pressing against her intestines.

Although I thought she might, Chris did not feel that her alternative therapies of vitamins, diet, and visualization had failed her. We talked about this in The Misery, the day after she was admitted. She had just learned that she had a new colon tumor.

"I've always accepted that I have a chronic and advanced disease," she said simply. "I've never expected a 'cure.' Maybe without the alternative therapies I've been practising, this would have happened sooner.

"Besides, I'm looking at it just as a lost battle," she said. "It's not the end of the war. Not by a long-shot!"

It was time for decisions again.

Robert Lotocki advised Chris that one option was to have the tumor removed surgically, followed by chemotherapy. As a chemotherapist, he clearly thought this was the route she should take. He had seemed disappointed when Chris had cut short her initial series of treatments. I got the impression that not only did he believe in chemotherapy as a possible 'cure' for Chris, but because he knew she was a fighter, he felt she was a good subject.

Lotocki was fair in advising her of the other option offered by conventional medicine. It was radiotherapy.

As always, we discussed it. I offered my opinion. She decided.

"I can't see myself going for another surgery," she said. "I barely survived the last one! And I just can't believe in chemo. It goes against everything that I feel is natural and positive, both mentally and physically." She thought a moment. "I may be wrong," she said. "But if I'm wrong, I'm wrong for me only. Nobody else will suffer the consequences."

She chose radiotherapy.

Chris's doctor in this was Kamalendu Malaker, who, like Lotocki, is associated with the Manitoba Cancer Treatment and Research Foundation. She was given a CAT-scan of the abdomen and pelvis to determine whether her situation was suitable for radiotherapy. The radiation oncologist from India concluded that it was. He also decided that her condition was critical and required immediate treatment.

The problem with this was the shortage of radiotherapy equipment. Chris said that Malaker seemed personally as well as professionally distressed when he told her that there were just a few units in the Manitoba health care system.

"I think he said three," Chris tried to recall. "And they're booked solid for weeks to come.

"He was quite candid that he didn't feel radiotherapy is being given equal billing with chemotherapy in cancer care in Manitoba," said Chris. "Apparently, it all depends on whether the person in charge is more inclined towards one or the other."

Dr. Malaker acted quickly and compassionately to get Chris the treatment that he considered critical. A phone call to Dr. Keith Arthur, Director of Radiotherapy, got her accepted at the Tom Baker Cancer Centre, in Calgary. Another, to the Director of the Manitoba Health Services Commission, arranged for a temporary transfer of health benefits. Malaker urged us to get going, while he prepared, for dispatch to Calgary, Chris's medical chart, her X-rays, and a covering letter.

He had told us that the series of radiation treatments, twenty-five in all, would take five weeks. We did not even consider staying with Casey and Elaine. We knew we would be welcome, but we had no idea how much the side effects from her radiation would affect Chris.

"Even if my reaction is mild," she said, "you can't parachute two people, one of them taking radiotherapy, into a young family with a fifteen-month-old child, for five weeks."

Chris had heard that when someone from out-of-town is undergoing lengthy treatment, the Canadian Cancer Society in some centres can provide hostel accommodation for the patient and their spouse. What we learned, beginning that day, is that the Canadian Cancer Society is not national in character, as the name suggests, but a collection of ten provincial jurisdictions.

I phoned the Canadian Cancer Society in Manitoba to ask about hostel accommodation in Calgary. It was a Friday afternoon.

"The person you need to speak to is not in," switchboard told me. "You have to call her either before noon on Fridays, or after noon on Mondays."

"That's a sweetheart of a job," said Chris.

I reached her after noon on Monday. It wasn't worth the wait. She had no information on hostel accommodation or any other services provided by the Canadian Cancer Society in Calgary. All she could tell me was the phone number. It was a relief when I called that number and got an enthusiastic, positive response.

"Yes, we've got hostel accommodation for your wife and yourself! You're arriving when? Thursday? Good! We'll arrange a courtesy room for the weekend at the Westin Hotel. Monday we'll get you into a hostel. What? No problem! Look forward to seeing you!"

I hung up. "Well, that was a breath of fresh air!" I said to Chris.

Little did we know.

We left Winnipeg by car two days later, a Wednesday in mid-October. As we had on the drive to the Olympics eight months earlier, we stopped over at the Journey's End Motel, in Swift Current. Going by car seemed like a good idea. For one thing, we would have to get Chris to her radiation treatment five days a week at the Tom Baker Cancer Centre. We might also be able to do a little family visiting and sightseeing.

Although we had been told that the side effects from radiation usually are not as severe as those from chemo, we still had no idea how Chris might react. Some patients are more affected than others.

"With luck," said Chris, "I might feel well enough on weekends for us to drive over to Casey and Elaine's. Maybe," she added a little wistfully, "we'll get back to Banff and Lake Louise."

It was not until the return trip that we realized that going by car, in one way, had been a mistake.

The Westin Hotel, on Fourth Avenue Southwest in downtown Calgary, is part of an international chain of luxury hotels and resorts that does something exceptional for cancer patients. It provides accommodation, at no charge, for those from out-of-town who are undergoing treatment. There are two riders: A vacant room has to be available. And the reservation must come from the Cancer Society. The policy was begun in 1982 when the Westin Hotel in Seattle, Washington, decided to do what it did best to assist visiting cancer patients. Since then, nineteen Westin Hotels in the United States, and three in Canada, have provided more than 25,000 courtesy rooms.

Chris, Nigel, and I got into Calgary early Thursday afternoon and checked in. We were given that broad western welcome that you expect from a hotel like the Calgary

Westin, and a large, comfortable room in The Tower, on the 18th floor.

I was busy unpacking our travel bag. Chris was checking out the view from our window. "Come look!" she called out.

You could see the sprawl of Calgary west, and beyond that the foothills of the Rockies. The first time I saw them, I was a wet-behind-the-ears reporter riding Canadian Pacific's "Dominion Limited " to the Coast, hoping to land a job with a Vancouver newspaper. I have loved those mountains ever since.

Not just as scenery. More like beckoning colossi, welcoming me into their own Brobdingnagian world. On the several drives that Chris and I made west from Calgary, my heart would start to quicken as the foothills loomed larger.

My wife knew how I felt.

Anyone listening in would have thought we were both quite mad.

"Can you hear them calling?" she would ask.

"Ohh, yes!" I would reply. "I can hear them. I can hear my mountains calling out to me!"

I really could. Just as importantly, Chris knew that I could. It was one of the wonderfully improbable secrets that we shared together.

I turned away from the view of the foothills and phoned the Cancer Society from our room. I was told that the woman I had spoken with when I called from Winnipeg was not available. I was asked to call back Monday. One o'clock Monday was our check-out time at the Westin.

Chris and I spent Friday and Saturday evening with Casey, Elaine, and our grandson. The rest of the time, she rested in our room, or we wandered around downtown Calgary. I knew that if there was one thing that would take her mind off her illness and help lift her spirits, it was browsing through the shops.

Monday dawned and I phoned the Canadian Cancer Society. I was told there was a problem. "We do have a nurses' residence that serves as a hostel," a young woman said hesitantly. "The fee is just nominal. The problem is, you and your wife aren't Albertans." There was a lengthy silence at both ends of the line. "The best we can do for you," the woman said finally, "is suggest a motel."

I asked to speak with the person I had spoken with by phone from Winnipeg: the enthusiastic, positive one who had said "Monday we'll get you into a hostel! No problem!"

There was another lengthy pause at the other end. "She's no longer with us."

Well, that's convenient. Just last Thursday Chris and I got a solid commitment from someone. Suddenly today, a week later, we're told that she's no longer a player.

I figured that at worst she probably got chewed out for not knowing the Society's "Albertans Only" rule.

"What's the name of the motel?" I asked.

The woman on the other end of the line sounded relieved. She gave me the name of a motel. I guess she felt that she should end on a positive note. "The Society recommends it," she said.

"Thanks," I said, and hung up.

Chris had heard enough from my end of the conversation to realize that something was wrong. "What is it?" she asked.

For more than thirty years, in Ontario and Manitoba, Chris and I had made donations at the office, at the house, and we always had bought Canadian Cancer Society daffodils.

"We bought all those damned daffodils," I said, "in the wrong provinces."

I made light of it on the drive to Motel Village in the northwest end of Calgary. "Staying at a motel will be like the old dog show days," I said.

Chris didn't reply. I could see she was upset. This rubbed off on me. Avoiding stress is one of the best ways to fight cancer, as well as to avoid it. When your cancer is critical and you've driven this distance, all the way psyching yourself up for five weeks of radiation, you don't need upset of any kind. She had been told to expect caring supportiveness from the Alberta arm of the national society that she had bought into all her life. Instead, she had been snubbed by a private members' club.

We pulled into the motel that the woman at the Cancer Society had recommended. While Chris sat in the car with Nigel, I entered the office. We needed a little kitchenette in case Chris was too tired, or too sick to go out, or if I had to cook up something special for her. I had brought from home the blender I used to make what she called her "power shakes."

I checked us in and the woman behind the counter gave me a stack of sheets and pillowcases. I thought this was a little odd, but I didn't say anything. The place had been recommended.

"Clean linens and cleaning once a week," she said.

I got into the car and drove us to our door. While Chris went inside with Nigel, I got our bags out of the trunk. When I entered, Chris was sitting on the edge of the bed. I remembered how her face fell when she saw the drab room in which she and another woman were to take chemotherapy. It hit rock bottom when she walked into this place that was to be her home for the next five weeks while she took radiation.

Someone had punched or kicked in one of the panels in

the door to the bathroom. It looked like a drink had been splashed on a wall. The bare mattress Chris was sitting on was soiled and sagging. The place was dirty.

I had never seen Chris look like she was about to give up. She still didn't. But she appeared to be perilously close. I dropped the bags and took her by the arm. "Come on," I said. "Let's get the hell out of here."

The woman in the motel office didn't look too surprised when I barged in, told her we'd had a change in plans, and asked for a refund. I guess I wasn't the first.

As the name suggests, there are plenty of places to stay in Motel Village. While Chris sat in the car, I drove from one to another, checked out the weekly rate for a room with kitchenette, and did a quick tour of the rooms. None of the motels was the disaster that the one recommended by the Cancer Society had been. They had to be passed up for other reasons. Some didn't have kitchenettes. Some were too pricy for a five-to-six-week stay. It was becoming late in the afternoon. I could see that Chris was getting wiped. On a hit-and-run of about the seventh motel, I found one that was acceptable.

The Panama Motor Inn, on Sixteenth Avenue Northwest, is owned and staffed by a family from East Africa. The room I took, with kitchenette, was spotless. There is daily maid service. The mattresses are Sealy Posturepedic. It is well-run and quiet. It is just a few steps from a Denny's Restaurant, which serves good food, reasonably priced, around the clock. It is close to a Safeway grocery store and Brentwood Mall.

I swear I saw Chris's eyes light up when I mentioned the mall!

The Panama Motor Inn also cost eight dollars a night less than the rat-trap that had been recommended by the Cancer Society.

I phoned the Society in the morning. I got the same

young woman I had spoken with the previous day. I asked her "Did anyone from the Cancer Society ever check out that motel you recommended? Did you or anyone else ever go there and look it over?"

She said that no one ever had.

"Then why would the Society recommend it?"

"The owners wrote us a letter," she said. "They said that they'd be happy to take cancer patients."

I hung up on the word "Incredible!"

It had begun with the uninformed long-weekender at the Society's Winnipeg office. Next had come the runaround in Calgary. Then the recommended motel that no one ever had bothered to check out. I had built up a good head of steam over the past few days. It lasted all the way back to Winnipeg.

I let it off in a letter to the Canadian Cancer Society's national headquarters, in Toronto. If they just had told us from the start that we were on our own, it would have been okay. What had upset Chris, which in turn served to infuriate me, were the empty assurances and bad advice that had led to her own unfulfilled expectations. I got a prompt response from the Society's national headquarters. Regretful and conciliatory, it included coverage of the cost of our motel.

Things had to get better, and they did.

The Tom Baker Cancer Centre is a confidence builder. Just a few minutes from the Panama Motor Inn, on Twenty-Ninth Street Northwest, it flanks Calgary's Foothills Hospital. The building itself is impressive—airy and modern, with a lively decor and the look of a florist's shop. It is the staff, though, from the Centre's medical people to its volunteer "tea ladies," that make it special.

Chris's romance with the Centre began on her first meeting with its director of radiotherapy, Dr. Keith Arthur. An affable Welshman, he ushered us into a room and we sat down. He put up Chris's CAT-scan, sent to him by Dr. Malaker, on a backlighted screen. Then he explained in layman's terms what we were looking at and what he hoped to accomplish. He gave it to us straight. I mentally thanked him for that. It was the way Chris always wanted it.

"Don't expect a cure," Arthur cautioned. He addressed Chris directly. "You have advanced cancer. In your case, we are looking at palliative radiation. By this I mean that our reasonable objectives are to halt the tumor's growth and shrink it. This will relieve the pressure on your vital organs, allowing them to function more normally. It also should decrease the pain and discomfort that you're feeling now."

"What side effects should I expect?" asked Chris.

"Weakness. Tiredness. Since we're radiating your lower abdomen, first feeling sick to your stomach, cramps. Then diarrhea later on. How severe these side effects are," Arthur added, "depends to a great degree on the individual. Different patients have lesser or greater reactions."

We talked a while longer about Chris's cancer and the Centre. Arthur said that they had little trouble getting first-rate staff because of the well-equipped facility itself. The proximity to great vacation and ski country. The climate, with its unexpectedly warming "chinooks" in winter. The Calgary "urban cowboy" lifestyle.

I could tell that Chris liked Keith Arthur. So did I.

Before we left, he made an appointment for Chris to visit the Simulator Room the next morning. We knew what this was from the comprehensive information packet, covering everything from radiation terms to diet, that the Centre provides when you register. The patient lies on a flat, narrow bed. Guided by diagnostic X-rays, the oncologist and the technologist establish the precise area to be radiated. The skin is marked with a marker pen.

"It shows them exactly where to radiate every time," Chris said. "So it's important not to wash the marks off."

Chris's first session was scheduled for the next morning. On the short drive to our motel, we stopped at the Safeway and picked up a few groceries. Because diarrhea is an almost certain side effect to radiation, usually after the first ten sessions or so, it is best to try to use diet against it from the start.

Chris had to cut out temporarily the high-fibre foods, like whole grain cereals and "roughage" fruits and vegetables, that she had been eating to help her stay healthy. These would contribute to diarrhea.

"At the same time," she said, "because my system has to rebuild itself after each radiation, I have to pump up on vitamins, proteins, and calories."

As well as the usual staples, we bought cheese, peanut butter, and a large box of skim milk powder. All are good sources of protein. I planned to spike Chris's "power shakes" with the skim milk powder, and sprinkle it over soups, the scrambled eggs she liked so much, even hamburger and pasta dishes.

Diarrhea weakens by dehydrating and draining off potassium. We laid in a lot of real fruit juice and bananas, as well as meat, fish, and potatoes. Bananas are not only high in potassium, but like block cheese, apple sauce, dry toast with peanut butter, and clear tea, they also help control diarrhea. Whether eating just across the way at Denny's or in our motel, Chris did her best each day to eat meat or fish, with potatoes or yams, and carrots or turnips.

The final purchase we made at Safeway was a box of Saran wrap. When she showered, Chris would wrap a length around her lower abdomen to keep the radiotherapy marks from being washed away.

There was an October nip in the air the next morning. I went out to the motel parking lot and got the car warmed up before Chris came out.

"Ready?" I asked, as she got into the car.

"As much as I'll ever be."

She had brought along a book to keep her mind occupied until it was time for her radiation. It was by the English-born Hollywood actress Jill Ireland, wife of Charles Bronson. Published just the year previous, it was the story of her battle with breast cancer since 1984, the same year that Chris had undergone surgery for colon cancer. Jill Ireland had had a radical mastectomy, which means that a breast, supporting fat and muscle, and fat and lymph nodes in the armpit had been amputated.

It sounds like a downer of a book for someone going into radiation, but Chris didn't see it like that. She empathized with Jill Ireland. She admired her for the gutsy way that she was facing her own life with cancer. In a sense, she felt that they were sisters.

As always, Chris looked for a little humor in her situation. A few years earlier, Charles Bronson had made a movie called *Death Wish*. The title Jill Ireland had given her book was *Life Wish*.

One of the teleplays I had written for "General Motors Presents," on CBC Network television, was called *The Radioactive Man*. As Chris and I entered the Centre for her first radiation, she said "Maybe when I tell my own story I should call it *The Radioactive Woman*!"

Actually, we had been told by Keith Arthur that radiation would not make her "radioactive." "There is no danger of this to the patient." he had said. "Nor is there any danger to anyone around them."

Chris and I sat down in one of the comfortable, off-corridor waiting-rooms in the radiotherapy section. We were greeted with a cheerful "Good morning!" by several other patients and their companions. The couple sitting next to us introduced themselves as being from Lethbridge, Alberta. The husband told us he was taking radiation for lung cancer.

We had ten minutes or so to wait until Chris's appointment. Two of the Centre's white-smocked "tea ladies" came up the corridor. They were pushing a cart with a silver tea and coffee service, china cups and saucers, cold drinks, paper napkins, and a tray of cakes and cookies.

While one of the volunteers gave us a choice of coffee, tea, milk, and fruit juices, the other passed around the tray of home-baking. I'm a freak for cookies, any kind of cookies. I picked an oatmeal one studded with chocolate chips.

"Go on!" the woman urged. "You're a big guy. Take two!"

"Don't encourage him!" Chris protested.

Her appointment was for 10:15.

Give or take a minute or two, her radiotherapy technologist came for her. The pleasant young woman in the white smock had the same upbeat manner as everyone else at the Centre, staff and patients alike. I squeezed Chris's hand and smiled my reassurance as she went with the technologist.

Chris told me after her first treatment, "There isn't really much to it."

Lying on a table in the radiation room, she was wheeled under a high-energy X-ray machine. When the technologist had positioned her, adjusting the machine to lock in on the marks that had been drawn on her abdomen, shields were set to protect the rest of her body. She was asked to lie still. The technologist exited to an adjacent control room. Chris was monitored visually and by intercom throughout. The actual treatment was over in a matter of minutes.

"All I got was a kind of warm feeling in the area being radiated," she said. "It's a little high-tech scary, though, your first time. I felt like doing the 'Star Trek' thing and calling out to my technologist: 'Beam me up, Scotty!'"

Other than being chronically tired, Chris didn't have any real problems the first couple or three weeks. She did a lot of cat-napping. The Panama Motor Inn has AM-FM radio and satellite television, so our evenings were spent pleasantly enough in the motel.

Weekends were "rest" days. Her treatments were suspended to give her body a break from the Monday-to-Friday bombardment it was taking. We dropped in frequently on Casey, Elaine, and our grandson. Going on one-and-a-half years, Tyson now was what Chris called "a little person," and much more fun to be with.

We also spent time browsing around Brentwood Mall, and did a little sightseeing by car, but we didn't go on any long drives. The radiation was making it progressively difficult for Chris to sit in one place for any length of time. She was finding that she had to keep changing position, or get up and walk around.

McMahon Stadium, home of the Calgary Stampeders of the Canadian Football League, was just a "Hail Mary" from our motel. Game nights, we could hear the roar of the crowd and look out our window at the stadium's canopy of floodlights. It was pretty obvious, though, that there was no way that Chris could sit through four quarters of football.

We did take one longer drive. We had heard how beautiful Kananaskis Provincial Park is, with its ice-capped mountains, glacier leftovers, lakes, and waterfalls. Shuttling daily between our motel and the Centre, we had the feeling that we were beginning to stagnate. We drove out one Sunday to see as much of the park as we could from the car and treat ourselves to dinner at Kananaskis Lodge.

Chris rose to the occasion. She fitted right in with the place, looking healthy and athletic in a bright yellow ski jacket. Her blonde hair had a windblown look. The cold mountain air brought color to her cheeks. I took a picture of her. She looked carefree and happy standing on the rim of the lodge's impressive, ice-coated water fountain. It was a good day.

The following week, Chris had an increase in the side effects from the radiation she was being given. She was more easily exhausted. She lost her appetite. She developed diarrhea. She was bothered by itching, where she was being radiated, that she was not allowed to scratch. She was finding it even more difficult to sit still for any length of time in one place or position.

I guess my concern showed.

"The Centre's being very supportive," Chris said reassuringly. "They're doing all they can for me."

I knew that she regularly had interviews with a therapist after her treatments. All I could do was be supportive in my own way. I tried to get her to eat regularly without bullying her. I cooked up soups and made "power shakes" laced with skim milk powder. I put together low-fibre snacks, like block cheese and crackers (not those processed yellow pasteboards) and peanut butter on dry white toast.

The first week in November, during a routine examination at the Centre, a lesion was discovered on Chris's scalp.

She was advised to have it looked at by a dermatologist.

"There's a procedure involved," Chris explained on the drive back to our motel. "First I have to go to my doctor, who'll refer me to a skin specialist. Since I haven't got a doctor here, I'll go to Casey's."

Casey was about as dynamically caring a son as any mother could hope for. He phoned his physician right away and asked for an immediate appointment. Dr. Colin Chandler saw Chris the next morning at his office in the Concept Health Clinic, in downtown Palliser Square.

"What's your problem?" he asked.

"I don't have a problem," Chris said, "I've got cancer."

I saw Chandler's eyebrows arch. Except for the chronic pallor that she camouflaged with the help of Estée Lauder, Chris most of the time looked remarkably well. It was on the inside that she was so devastatingly ill. "You look fine to me," Chandler said.

He examined the lesion. Then he got on the phone and arranged an early appointment with a dermatologist. As we were leaving, he said to Chris "Well, if you say you've got cancer I guess you have. Good luck to you."

The dermatologist Chandler referred Chris to was Dr. Howard Cohen, at the Mission Professional Centre. He looked at the lesion in her scalp and said it was "just a sign of old age."

Later, when we were talking about it, Chris said "An Italian doctor would have said it better!"

Cohen told her that he could burn it off, but would rather not. He said he didn't want to cause her any more discomfort than she already was having from radiation.

"Almost an afterthought," Chris said, "I asked him to look at that mole on the back of my shoulder."

This was a "beauty mark" that she had had from childhood. Over the past while, it had seemed to her that it was becoming larger. The dermatologist examined it.

"How long have you had this?" Without waiting for Chris to reply, he said "This is what we should be looking at."

He wondered out loud why she hadn't noticed it before now. "More to the point," he said, "I wonder why none of your doctors did. Somebody should have."

"I guess they were too busy at the other end," Chris said.

"And you just noticed it recently? You're not very observant either."

"I've also been pretty busy at the other end."

Dr. Cohen took a small slice of the mole to send to a lab for a biopsy. He was concerned that Chris had a relatively rare type of melanoma, or cancer of the skin. It spreads quickly, usually to vital organs like the lungs, liver, and brain, which makes it particularly lethal. At most danger are light-skinned people who have been overexposed to the sun.

Chris, my green-eyed, blonde, fair-skinned Aztec, had been a sun worshipper all her life.

"As a teen-ager spending my summers at 'Ramona,'" she had once told me, "I would lie near-naked by the hour on the roof of the boathouse. In winter, in my bedroom, I sometimes fell asleep under one of those old-fashioned sun-lamps. More than once, I woke up looking like a cooked lobster!"

She didn't have to go back that far. I remembered that Chris had spent much of our summers working on a tan in Muskoka, when we lived in Toronto, and at Victoria Beach, on Lake Winnipeg. On a couple of winter vacations we had taken, she had chased the sun south to Florida.

Brown was beautiful.

We didn't discuss any of this, or the possible results of the biopsy, over the weekend. It was just too much to speculate on whether it would show that Chris had been stricken by a third cancer. Possibly the most lethal one of all.

My God! She's still being treated for a return of the first and second ones! How much can she cope with?

I got my answer shortly after 9:15 a.m. Monday, when we had left Dr. Cohen's office. He had advised us that the mole was malignant. Because that type of melanoma can spread so rapidly, with such deadly results, he had booked Chris for surgery at 2:30 p.m. that same day.

Outside the office, I didn't know what to say. Or if I should say anything. What *could* I say?

I guess Chris knew what was going through my mind. She tucked her arm in mine. "Okay," she said. "So it's three strikes. *But not out!*"

I wondered how many people could have handled it that well. I know I couldn't have. She told me later that the visualization she had been practising was a big factor. "It gives me a communication with my body that gives me confidence in its ability to fight back," she said, "no matter what. When we got back to the motel, I had a talk with my inner self. I told the cells in the white hats, 'Well, you screwed up pretty good on the skin thing!' And they said, 'Hang in there, lady. Remember that it ain't over 'til it's over!'"

Dr. Frank Sutton, a specialist skilled in cancer surgery, met us at Colonel Belcher Hospital, not far from his office at the Rideau Medical-Dental Centre, on Fourth Street Southwest. He cut out the mole and some of the surrounding tissue. The lab pathologist had staged Chris's melanoma as 1B, or Clarke's III.

This is the second stage. It meant that the malignant growth had reached a depth of between .76 and 1.5 millimetres. The surgery took just a few minutes. It was an important few minutes.

Frank Sutton's parting remark, referring both to his surgery and Howard Cohen's spot diagnosis, was "We just saved your life."

Chris and I showed up the next day at 10:30 a.m., at the Tom Baker Cancer Centre, for her radiation treatment. Keith Arthur suggested that because of her surgery for melanoma, the radiation treatments be laid off for a week. Despite the problems, from chronic hurting to weariness to diarrhea that she was having, Chris asked that they proceed. "If it's going to do any good," she said, "let's get it over with."

Chris was one tough lady.

How I admired her for that!

Her radiation treatments at the Tom Baker Cancer Centre ended the last week in November. She rested up for a couple of days, and we spent our last evening in Calgary with Casey, Elaine, and Tyson. We both knew that the drive home was going to be a problem. As her radiation treatments had progressed, so had the itching and aching in her lower abdomen. Because of this, she was almost continually getting up and moving around in our motel. I figured that the two-day drive from Calgary back to Winnipeg might be next to intolerable.

I suggested that she fly while I drove.

"No."

"Why not?"

"Who would look after you?"

The first mistake we had made was choosing to come by car, although I don't know what we would have done without one. The second was our decision to go home by way of Montana. Chris did not like the prospect of driving through the monotonous flatlands of eastern Alberta, Saskatchewan, and Manitoba. We had made that trip too many times.

We decided to drive south of Calgary into Montana, east to North Dakota, then north to Winnipeg. It was not all that much farther. Besides, I thought a route we'd never driven before might help take Chris's mind off the itching and aching in her lower abdomen. She was having soreness, too, where the surgeon had exorcised the cancer in her shoulder.

We didn't realize that the route south into Montana is mountainous and it was well into winter in the mountains.

The first couple of hours was a pleasant drive. It was November 27, Grey Cup Day. On our car radio, the Winnipeg Blue Bombers were playing a close game against the British Columbia Lions. Then the road began a steep climb and we drove into a snowstorm. We lost radio reception. (We heard when we got home that Winnipeg had squeaked out a 22-21 win.)

The region we were driving through is summer vacation country. Everything, including motels and all but one gas station, was closed for the season. The road was winding and treacherous, with hairpin curves that looked out over eternity. On many of these, there were one or more simple wooden crosses.

I was trying very hard to see through my snowy windshield and anticipate those curves. On a drive like this, I thought our survival kit should have included a couple of parachutes.

"What are those crosses for?" Chris asked.

The driving really was tough going. I knew she was hurting, wriggling around in the seat, trying to get comfortable for even a few minutes at a time. She didn't need any more stress than she already had.

"I guess they're sort of roadside shrines," I said, straining to keep the car on track. We entered an abrupt, L-shaped turn in the road that had five of the little crosses planted on the lip of the invisible gorge below.

Chris looked at them as I did a tight wheel, then back at me as I straightened the car out again. "My God!" she said. "Those crosses are for people who've been killed on these curves!"

I told her the crosses were put there by the Montana department of highways as a warning to people to drive safely. "Don't worry," I said. "None of them have our names on them."

Chris was silent for the rest of the drive through the mountains. We both were relieved when we left the mountain-goat curves and the snowstorm behind us and got down into the valley. All I wanted was to get Chris out of this car and into a motel, so she could make herself a little more comfortable. I floored it and sped through the Montana black. Within a matter of a few minutes, I caught the reflection of flashing roof-lights in my rear-view mirror.

Chris looked over her shoulder. "Oh-Oh," she said.

"Yeah," I agreed.

I pulled over.

The young guy who got out of the Montana Highway Patrol car looked like a stand-in for John Wayne. He was tall and slim, with one of those Stetson hats and what I assumed was a Colt .45 slung at his side in a leather holster.

Cancer puts a lot of continuing strain on the spouse of the person who has it. It is stressful, too, for the rest of the family and for friends. It comes from your love and concern for the patient. That and an enduring feeling of frustration. Of helplessness. You try not to let it show. The person with cancer has enough problems without feeling guilty about stressing out their family and friends.

After that nerve-wracking all-day drive, Chris's five weeks in radiation, then learning that she had melanoma, knowing how scared and hurting she was, and staying brave about it, I had had it. I got out of the car and met the highway patrolman halfway. I guess I looked like I was ready for the Gunfight at the OK Corral.

"Okay," I said. "So I was speeding. I have a damn good reason!"

He was already writing out the ticket. "What's the reason?"

"My wife just took five weeks of radiation for cancer in Calgary. I have to get her off the road. Give me the damn ticket and tell me how far it is to the nearest motel."

John Wayne stopped writing and studied me a moment. Then he closed his book and gestured down the highway. "About twenty minutes," he said. "Drive carefully."

I was told at the motel that the Highway Patrol, like the Mounties, have a tradition. The Mounties always get their man. The Montana Highway Patrol never tears up a speeding ticket.

If you read this, John Wayne, thank you.

Because it was easier on Chris, we pulled off the road early the next afternoon and checked into another motel. On the third day of what is usually a two-day drive, we arrived home.

The reaction to the radiation wore off in a week or so and Chris got back into her regular regime of diet, vitamins, visualization, and "jalking." There was no doubt that the radiation had done what it was supposed to do. The obstructing tumor had been shrunk to the point that it was no longer a problem. Her stomach had stopped swelling.

Over the next couple of weeks, Chris threw herself into gift-shopping, wrapping, decorating the house, and doing her best to fill it with Christmas trees. My big job, as it was every year, was trying to fit a ten-foot tree that was "too small" into a dining-room with a nine-foot ceiling.

Chris had thought of going on from Calgary to the Hope Cancer Health Centre, in Vancouver. "We'll be halfway there," she reasoned. She dropped that idea when it became obvious that she couldn't sit in the car all the way out to the Coast and back. It proved to be tough enough for her just to make it home.

Hope was the first centre in Canada to offer cancer patients visualization workshops. The Centre was founded in 1980 by Claude Dosdall, the man who wrote the book *My God, I Thought You'd Died!*, and is staffed by people with cancer.

Dosdall himself was diagnosed with an inoperable brain tumor in 1977. He confounded the medical professionals by living a good many years beyond what they had predicted. His neurosurgeon had told him that he possibly had one— at the most five—years to live. He died sixteen years later, in 1993.

When Dosdall appeared on the "Oprah Winfrey Show," he told Oprah and her viewers that his philosophy was simple: If you eat properly, exercise, and think yourself well, you can make yourself well. Or at least a little better.

With Christmas behind us, it was time for New Year's resolutions. Chris didn't have to tell me hers. I knew that she was resolved, early in the coming year, to get to the Hope Cancer Health Centre.

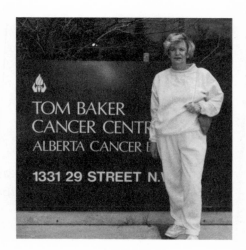

Tom Baker Cancer Centre. Calgary. Fall '88 — The Centre is impressive, but it's the staff, from medical team to 'tea ladies' who make it special.

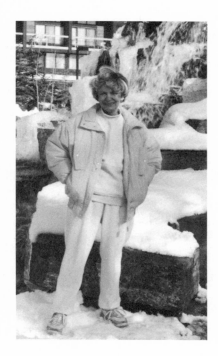

A day off from radiation. Kananaskis, Alberta. Fall '88 — Her blonde hair had a wind-blown look. The mountain air brought color to her cheeks. She looked carefree and happy.

8·Looking good, living well

As it turned out, Chris was to keep her New Year's resolution in mid-March.

Late in January, she ferreted out a reasonable, pre-booked travel package that provided us with our flight, a week at a luxury hotel and a U-drive in Vancouver.

Over the winter, Dr. McIntyre had begun making twice-weekly house calls. He would ask Chris how she felt and listen to any questions or comments either of us had about her condition. He dropped by after his early hospital rounds at The Misery, usually by about 8:00 a.m.

His arrival at our place was a production. Don McIntyre was not into parallel parking. I would clear a runway for him by arrangement with my co-operative neighbors on both sides. Just before his arrival, three car spaces hastily would be cleared. A few minutes later, Dr. McIntyre would bring in his white Jaguar like he was landing a Boeing 737 at Winnipeg International Airport.

Before leaving, he would inject Chris with Vitamin B1. He admitted it was controversial, like all vitamin therapy, but he believed in it. "At the very least," Dr. McIntyre said, "I think it's an effective 'picker-upper.'"

Chris had built a good deal of hedonism into our visit to the coast for the cancer workshop. A cousin of mine generously had offered a month's loan of his vacant ocean-side house on Vancouver Island. After that, Chris had arranged a trip with a friend down the Oregon Coast to the Planetree Health Resource Center, in San Francisco, then on to California's Big Sur country.

The day before we left, McIntyre provided us with enough bottled Vitamin B1 and disposable hypodermic needles to last Chris until our return. He showed me how to use them. It was my first experience at learning to be a sort of paramedic to my wife. It would turn out, in time, to be just the beginning.

Our registration at the Hope Cancer Health Centre had been confirmed in a letter from the Centre's Maggie Vance in late February. A couple of weeks later, Chris, Nigel, and I flew Air Canada to the Coast two days early. We picked up our U-drive at the airport and checked into the Bayshore Westin, on West Georgia Street.

The Bayshore, with Edmonton's Westin Hotel and the Calgary Westin, make up the three members of the chain in Canada that provide out-of-town cancer patients with courtesy accommodations. The program applies only to those undergoing conventional medical treatment.

Our introductory session at the Centre was Friday evening. The actual working part of the workshop would take place over Saturday and Sunday.

"Let's be tourists!" Chris said.

It wasn't a hard game to play. We've always been lucky with rooms-with-a-view. This one made picture postcards of the mountains, the ocean and the Vancouver skyline. Beneath lay the harbor and hotel marina, with their odd contrast of lazy sailboats and hurry-up seaplanes. Cooper Air, from Vancouver Island, other chartered and scheduled flights, and private planes come and go as regularly as taxis.

"Has it changed much since you lived here?" Chris wanted to know.

"Unbelievably!" I replied. "When I worked on *The Province*, Vancouver was a small town with big city ambitions. In about fifty years," I gestured towards the skyline, "just look."

"Impressive," Chris said.

"Yes. But I wonder how much nostalgia there is for the way it was."

Over the next couple of days, we rediscovered some of Vancouver's past in walks through historic Gastown and a drive through Stanley Park. When I first came to Vancouver, someone told me "It wasn't worth logging. They didn't know what else to do with it. So they threw a fence around it and called it a park." I'm sure the story is apocryphal, but everyone who visits this natural ocean-front thousand acres comes away glad that it was left untouched.

The seawall is a jogger's paradise. The paths through the park are a stroller's. We parked the car and walked for a while, stopping to have lunch in a quaint English setting in the Teahouse Restaurant, at Ferguson Point.

Based on the most optimistic prognosis given him by his neurosurgeon, Claude Dosdall had been dead four years when he welcomed Chris and me on Friday evening to the Hope Cancer Health Centre, a storefront conversion on West Broadway. The Centre's founder was a wiry, kinetic person with an immediate impact: You knew right away that he had a keen interest in staying alive, and in helping others do the same.

Beginning with Dosdall, everyone in the room, except for companions like myself, had cancer.

Altogether, along with Dosdall and three or four staff members, there were about two dozen of us. There was no gloom and doom. Quite the opposite. A tape machine was playing Bobby McFerrin's catchy, bouncy "Don't Worry, Be Happy!" We were all milling about, introducing ourselves to each other. Laughing and talking. Maybe a little self-consciously. Maybe a little uncertainly, not knowing what to expect from the workshop that would start next morning.

It was odd. Until just a few minutes earlier, we had been strangers. Now we no longer were. We had discovered a profound and common bond. We all had cancer, or were with someone we loved who did. As Chris had felt like a sister to Jill Ireland, after reading *Life Wish*, we all now experienced this same sense of family. Just two days later, when the workshop broke up on Sunday evening, we hugged each other, chastely and naturally, like loving brothers and sisters.

I was reminded then of the words of Bernie Siegel, the New Haven, Connecticut, surgeon Chris had quoted to me: "Love heals!"

Now, Dosdall called our group to order. He welcomed us and told us what to expect. There would be a group therapy session just for those with cancer. Another just for their spouses. And still another, the final one, that would bring both together. He would lead structured visualization sessions daily. We were advised to wear something comfortable. Those who wanted to could bring a pillow or a blanket. There would be an hour-and-a-half lunch break. We could choose from several recommended restaurants nearby, including one for vegetarians.

Dosdall had just finished telling us this when the door

opened and a latecomer entered. He was a young man, late twenties or early thirties, with what was then called the "yuppie" look ("young, upwardly mobile business person"). He had two younger women with him. I guessed that one was his wife, the other a sister. Or maybe both were sisters. They found seats together on a sofa while Dosdall did a brief summation of what he had just finished telling the rest of us.

The newcomer had brought his own closed space with him. While his two companions whispered and smiled their hellos, he hardly looked around him, let alone spoke to anyone.

He was so uptight, it rubbed off. I felt sorry for him. At the same time, he made me a little uneasy. I didn't think I was the only one.

He didn't last through the Saturday session. At a break in the group therapies, we were all sitting or standing around, having coffee and talking. He and his two women companions were a closed trio again on the sofa. Abruptly, he stood up.

"This isn't going to help me!" Although he spoke in a loud voice, he seemed to be talking only to himself. "This won't do me any good! It's a waste of my time!"

As he spoke, he was throwing his coat over his shoulders. The room had fallen silent. One of the women got up, put her arm around him, and tried to soothe him with soft hushes. He shook her off. The other woman looked embarrassed enough for all three of them. She bowed her head as they followed the man quickly across the floor and out into the street.

Faith in anything, perhaps particularly in self, is not easy. There was a lengthy, awkward silence. A few moments of self-doubt so tangible it was reflected in people's faces. Then it passed.

Someone, I guess a staff member, put Bobby McFerrin back on the tape machine. The incident, as sad as it was for the man who couldn't believe in himself, was lost in the music and a return to conversation.

I was proud of Chris and everyone else in that room who had cancer. We had just seen how it can pull the rug out from under someone. It was apparent that come what may, they weren't going to let that happen to them. They were the survivalists.

It's remarkable how individual we all think we are, when in fact we basically are so very much alike. While Chris and the others with cancer were at their own group therapy session in another room, we husbands and wives were holding ours. Our moderator was a very warm and empathetic woman named Barbara Dans. She had heard it all before.

It came my turn to tell on myself. I recounted the incident with the vacuum cleaner, when I had tried to take it away from Chris.

"It was just after her colon surgery," I said sheepishly. "I was just trying to make sure she didn't overdo it."

Everybody at the table broke up. Practically in a chorus they admitted to making the same mistake, if not in precisely the same way, of being overprotective. With one husband, it actually had been over a vacuum cleaner. A wife had wound up arm-wrestling with her husband when he resented her insistence on helping him up and down stairs. Some of us had been stressing out our spouses by never talking about cancer. Others by talking about it too much.

It came down to striking a balance; to realizing that while cancer is a fact of our own and our spouse's lives, it is not the only, or even the most important fact.

Our group agreed that the cancer patient's spouse should

learn enough about the disease to be able to discuss it intelligently. We should talk about it when he or she wants to talk about it, openly and casually. We should advise our family and friends to do the same.

When it comes to physical assistance, we should be sure that our spouse needs and wants our help.

"You don't grasp the arm of a sightless person crossing the street," someone said. "You let them take yours."

It was suggested that we show the person with cancer the same consideration.

While we were discussing this, I remembered thinking, not long after Chris's colon surgery: *How can she find out what her limits are without testing them?*

Chris's cancer group had discussed pretty much the same problems, but with a reverse perspective. We talked about it over luncheon at the vegetarian restaurant. Neither of us was an all-out vegetarian, but the meat-free menu seemed to fit the mood of the weekend.

Chris pulled my leg a little. "I'm to realize that you might act dumb sometimes!" she said. Then seriously: "The consensus we reached is that problems, whatever they are, have to be brought out into the open and discussed frankly."

I recalled problems we had resolved by talking them out. One was when the uneaten food I had cooked for Chris landed in the garbage can, and I looked upon it as a case of unrequited love. Then there were the cooking odors, when she was taking chemotherapy, that I was unaware made her nauseated. I remembered how, first by frowning, then by coming right out with it, she had let me know how much she resented my being overprotective.

Chris and I never had had any difficulty discussing her cancer. Because I had sat in from the start on her consultations with doctors, I always knew her situation as fully as she did. She had kept me advised of her research on cancer. Then on its conventional medical treatment. After that, on alternative therapies. We always had talked openly about these things. But inability or unwillingness to communicate emerged as a major problem with some of the couples at the workshop.

It all came together the next day at the group therapy mixed session. All the major points that those with cancer had made among themselves, and that we had made among ourselves, were tossed on the table.

Couples who had experienced problems breaking down the talk barrier didn't have any now. Bottled-up insecurities and resentments popped out like genies.

It sometimes may have seemed like a spirited but good-natured free-for-all, with Barbara Dans acting more as referee than moderator, but it worked. We all came away with much more confidence about how, both individually and as couples, to deal with this disease that had invaded our lives.

The Centre's founder had led our first visualization session the previous day. We all sat, eyes closed, while a staff member started the tape machine. The music that Dosdall used as background for his soft, measured monologue was baroque: Pachelbel's "Canon."

With some personal variations, all visualization therapy is based on the Simonton technique. This, in turn, is rooted in principle and style to techniques of self-awareness and spiritual enrichment originated by the ancients of various cultures. The Hindu system of yoga is the most familiar example.

I won't try to repeat Dosdall's monologue. Just the framework. The words wouldn't come off that well without his own delivery and the Pachelbel staging, and they're a little different each time anyway.

He began with the suggestion that we relax by fixing our minds on our breathing. Think of nothing but "inhale" and "exhale." This makes you fully and precisely conscious of your body.

Then think of your cancer. See it as weak and deformed cells. To create the energy to reinforce that belief, make a fist. Relax it and think of your white cells. See them as programmed to seek out and destroy the cancer cells.

Go with them. They know exactly what to do. All they need from you is energy. Provide it for them by clenching your fist again. Relax it as you see them destroy the cancer cells.

Think of your life as being guided by the Universe, just as your white cells are. Let your mind take you to somewhere beautiful and restful. Relax there. Realize that the Universe wants you to be healthy and happy. Open yourself to its help.

The workshop ended after this last visualization session. After all the hugging and goodbyes were over, Chris and I went back to the Bayshore. Because we knew it was unlikely that we ever would see any of these couples again, we felt a sense of loss. We had spent only the workshop weekend together, but for those two days, in a very positive and special way, we all had become "friends for life."

Ivy Mason's late husband, Don, had been city editor when I was a reporter on *The Province* in Vancouver. Our families had become friends some years later, when Don went into high-powered public relations, the Masons moved to Toronto, and I was on the editorial staff of *The Telegram*. Ivy was living in White Rock. She had remarried and again been widowed.

She picked us up by car at the Bayshore and we ferried from Tsawwassen through the picturesque Gulf Islands to Sidney. My cousin Walter King, and his wife Brigitte, were not long out from Montreal. They had bought a beautiful home on an ocean inlet, just a few minutes from the Sidney ferry terminal, not far from the town itself.

Wally and his wife were planning a month's vacation back east. When they heard that we were visiting the Hope Centre in Vancouver, they offered us their house for a month.

It was a wonderful four weeks. Chris and I didn't understand then, and I still don't, why anyone would want to vacation off Vancouver Island. "There's everything here," she said. "Mountains. Ocean. Climate. Great people. World-class shopping. Why go anywhere else?" She loved the magnificent drive up the Malahat from Victoria north to Parksville. Then west to the still white sands and restless surf of Long Beach, in Pacific Rim National Park.

At the end of our month at Wally and Brigitte's, we rejoined Ivy Mason for a drive down the rugged Oregon coast to San Francisco. Chris wanted to visit the Planetree Health Resource Center, on Webster Street. This was the Center that had provided us with a printout of the latest computerized information on the treatment and prognosis for all stages of ovarian cancer. Its library is open to the public. Chris spent an hour or so seeking to up-date the information she had been sent a couple of years earlier.

"There's nothing new," she reported. She wasn't dispirited. She hadn't expected there would be.

Hedonism. We enjoyed the cable cars and Fisherman's Wharf. Chris had a glass of white wine and I had a couple of Michelobs during the "happy hour" in the penthouse piano bar of our Holiday Inn. We both found it a little eerie, looking out over San Francisco Bay at the empty tomb of Alcatraz. In the downtown shopping district, we were shocked to see so many street people begging for money. The saddest was a vacant-eyed young woman squatting outside the entrance to Macy's upscale department store. She was hugging a teddy bear.

From San Francisco, we took another great drive down the California coast for a week's stay in Carmel, with a side trip to the steep cliffs and savage surf of Big Sur. At the end of April, we parted company with Ivy in White Rock and flew back to Winnipeg.

The final adventure was Nigel's. He was missing when we landed. A computer check by Air Cargo revealed that someone had fouled up and off-loaded him in his crate at Saskatoon. Air Canada put him on the next flight east. An anxious Chris and I waited up for him until well past midnight. She needn't have worried. He arrived at the house, unruffled and in style, in an airport limousine.

Into late spring and through the summer, Chris managed to continue looking good and living well. She had periodic bowel problems and some swelling of her stomach, "but nothing," as she put it, "that I can't handle."

June had marked another sweet victory in her war with cancer. Chris had been determined to live to see her first grandson, born two years earlier. Casey and Elaine since had moved from Calgary to the Coast. Her second grandson, Colin, a brother for Tyson, had been born on June 10, in Vancouver's Shaughnessy Hospital. We didn't know it yet, but Casey and Elaine already were planning to bring the two children home to their grandmother's for Christmas.

In August, we took a cottage for a couple of weeks at Victoria Beach, about an hour's drive north on Lake Winnipeg. Every summer since returning to Manitoba, we had rented a place either at "the Lake," or "the Beach." Every Winnipegger knows that "the Lake" is Lake of the Woods, where Chris's family had once had their island cottage, and "the Beach" is Victoria Beach.

Victoria Beach is summer charm in a time warp. Most of the cottages are old and rambling, with screened porches and posted names like "The Hempsteads' Hideaway" or "Suits Us!" Strolling by, you might hear Big Band music on acetate 78s, from the 1930s and 40s, being played on a porch gramophone. A few vintage cottagers still fly the Union Jack on painted sapling flagpoles. There are no restaurants or bars. In season, no cars are permitted. Everybody walks, bikes, or goes by Beach taxi. This and the unbroken peace are enforced by the summer municipality's own police force.

We had a good friend there named Alice Grover. We would spend our days swimming and sunning on the warm white sands of Manitoba's freshwater sea. In the evening, we would return as voyeurs of sunsets so passionate the whole horizon blushed.

Being at "the Beach" gave Chris a lot of pleasure that summer. It was not until Thanksgiving that intestinal pain and chronic diarrhea suggested a recurrence of her colon cancer. She made an appointment with Don McIntyre. She didn't say anything until after we had left his office in the Medical Arts Building and were standing waiting for the elevator.

"Dr. McIntyre did a rectal," she said.

I knew from the way she said it what was coming next.

"He found another tumor."

McIntyre had made an appointment for Chris to see Arnold Rogers the next day. Rogers confirmed that Chris had a large tumor in her colon. Both McIntyre and he advised against further surgery. It would be followed by chemotherapy.

"They both know I'd never agree to chemo."

"So what do they suggest?"

"Perhaps more radiation. Or maybe just medication and a special diet."

It was six years since Arnold Rogers had stunned us with the news that Chris had colon cancer. I remembered that we had walked down the stairs in the Doctors' Building and stood at the entrance, sorting out our feelings. Just as we were doing now.

Chris looked a little rueful. "I get the impression that I'm running out of options," she said.

Bill and Gerrie Morriss had asked us to drop by after Chris's appointment. We did. The Morrisses are gracious hosts and good conversationalists. I had a Scotch. Chris had a sherry. I don't remember what we talked about.

All I can recall between Arnold Rogers' office and the drive home was thinking *My God! Does it never end? Knowing, as Chris did, that with most cancers it never does.*

Chris knew she was fortunate. She had won her personal war with cancer for six good years. Others, from personal friends to public figures, had not been so successful.

When Chris had been doing advertising and promotion for Eaton's, she had worked with a beautiful young model named Cheryl Lee. They had become friends. Just last August, Cheryl had been told that she had cancer. Chris was shocked the last week in October to read that she had died, just three months later.

Chris had been reading *It's Always Something* by Gilda Radner. This is the poignant, sometimes funny story of the television comedian's attempts to cope with ovarian cancer. She had died the previous spring, before her book got into print.

There were so many others. Particularly friends, like John Livingston, who had been one of the artists at Eaton's. Nancy McLaughlin, who had shown Dalmatians in our Group 6 at the dog shows. So many friends and friends of friends.

Casey, Elaine, and the children flew in from the Coast and made Christmas memorable for all of us. We had a dozen or so family, friends, and neighbors in for an old-fashioned rum eggnog party. (The secret is to use a quality dark rum, add a splash of bourbon, refrigerate the eggnog overnight, and fold the whipped whites in separately.) I contributed this and my "Un-Christmas Cake," thick with fruits held together by the barest of batters. Over the past few Christmases, this had become such a favorite that we now gift-wrapped it for family and friends.

Chris laid out a buffet of her own baking: plenty of seasonal tarts and cookies, tasty hors d'oeuvres, and two large spinach quiches that went fast, proving that real men *do* eat quiche!

New Year's Eve we spent with our good neighbors, the Prudens. As well as a great buffet, the Prudens provide a Pickwickian twist to seeing in the New Year. Gordon, a non-drinker, recreated an Old English tavern in his basement. He and his wife, Eileen, furnished it with pub trappings brought back from vacations overseas. Everything is authentic, except that I don't ever recall hearing Gordon call out "Time, gentlemen!"

It was not long after New Year's that Don McIntyre, on one of his regular weekly house calls, suggested to Chris that she consider laser treatment. Put simply, he said that the tumor is burned off by a precisely directed laser beam. In a similar treatment, called photodynamic therapy, tumor-destructive chemicals are activated by a beam of light.

"Laser has been found effective in clearing tumor-blocked organs," he said. "It's especially useful for treating patients who might have problems with further surgery."

McIntyre said that if Chris agreed to try laser treatment, he would contact Dr. Hartley Stern, at Toronto's Mount Sinai Hospital.

"Stern is a gynecological oncologist surgeon from Bethesda." he said.

He was referring to Bethesda Naval Hospital, in Maryland. It has one of the leading cancer treatment programs in the United States. For the past twenty years or so, it consistently has been endorsed by the American College of Surgeons' Commission on Cancer.

Chris and I discussed it after Don left. Chris had the final word. "Cancer as advanced as mine," she said, "is the Grand Master. I know that eventually it will say 'checkmate!' But before that happens, I intend to make all the moves open to me."

There was no underlying hysteria. No wringing of hands. No self-pity. It was a simple statement of fact, as she saw and accepted it.

In Toronto, at Mount Sinai in February, she was told that she could not be considered a candidate either for laser or photodynamics. Her tumor was on the inside wall of the intestine. It could not be treated without damaging adjacent organs.

Dr. Stern referred her to Dr. Joan Murphy, also a well-respected gynecologist oncologist surgeon, at Toronto General

Hospital. Murphy recommended that she do a laparotomy. This is exploratory surgery of the abdomen to find out how widespread the cancer is and what, if anything, can be done about it.

Nothing could be.

"The tumor is too large, extending into the pelvis," Dr. Murphy said. "It's also quite fixed. I was afraid that if I attempted to cut it out, your wife would bleed to death."

Chris had no choice now but her alternative therapies.

We practised visualization together in the morning and evening. She continued both her diet and vitamin therapies. She could no longer "jalk," but we took frequent casual walks over not-too-long distances.

It was a shock to Chris when Jill Ireland died in May. She read about Ireland's death in the newspaper. I could see that it troubled her. The Hollywood star had fought a much-publicized series of battles with cancer of the breast. It finally had metastasized to the liver and bones.

That evening, Chris got out *Life Wish* and re-read some of the passages she liked best. It was not until it was time for bed that she put it down. "Jill Ireland fought cancer for six years," she said. "All that time, Charles Bronson was her life support." She took my arm. "Just as you are mine."

One of the points Jill makes in her book, and Chris picked up on, was her interest in crystals. Some people believe that certain minerals have special powers, just as some believe that pyramids do.

The large chunk of blue crystal that Chris placed on our coffee table was hematite in amethyst. It had been mined in Thunder Bay, Ontario, and sent to Chris by her sister-in-law, Diana. The small stones that she collected were rose quartz, turquoise, and bloodstone. She wore them in a small, soft leather pouch around her neck, along with a pyramid-shaped quartz point.

I don't know about Jill Ireland, but I don't think Chris ever actually attributed healing powers to these stones that became special to her. I think she just saw them as mementos of creation, inspiring her to endure. And she loved beautiful things.

That summer, we again rented a cottage at Victoria Beach. In previous years, we sometimes bicycled to the bake shop to sneak a couple of forbidden cinnamon buns, fresh out of the oven. Now I went alone for them, while Chris waited back at the cottage. She had tried riding one of the bicycles that come with most cottages at "the Beach," but had found it too difficult.

One very clear evening, we walked down to Sunset Drive, the dirt road that rims the cottages by the lakeshore, and watched the sun go down. Chris got so much enjoyment from this, I thought that cancer perhaps had given her new insights into herself and the world around her. In the gathering dusk, on one of our slow strolls back to the cottage, I asked her about this.

"I wish I could say that having cancer had 'made me look at life in a new way,'" she said, "as some cancer patients do. It hasn't. I'm more conscious of how good it is to be alive. I appreciate the natural beauty around me more. I'm nicer to myself. Beyond that, cancer hasn't changed me or my perceptions."

"I have heard some say, 'Cancer has taught me so much.'"

"Whatever it has taught these people," Chris said, "I can do without. All it has taught me is that I'd rather not have it."

Cancer in someone you love throws a long shadow of guilt. In the beginning I had felt guilty because Chris had been stricken instead of me. I had worried over whether I was not doing enough for her. Or too much. Then I was concerned that I may have helped persuade her to make decisions she shouldn't have.

Now I felt guilty that I wasn't wealthy. I couldn't get her to one of those exclusive little foreign clinics that you hear work miracles. Then it dawned on me that this didn't make sense. People with so much money it's spilling out of their suitcases can't buy fly-in cures. There is no Shangri-La for advanced cancer patients.

Chris's symptoms, and the discomfort and pain that accompanied them, came, went, and came back again. Arnold Rogers periodically examined her and prescribed medicine. Don McIntyre kept up his weekly house calls. I think even more than the Vitamin B1 shots, the gentle and positive dialogues that he held with Chris were her best "picker-uppers."

This Christmas was much quieter than the previous one, when the grandchildren had come to visit. We still did the trees and "decked the house with boughs of holly," but because Chris didn't feel up to it, the decorating was left up to me. This was a departure from family tradition. I belonged to the "icicle toss" school of tree dressers. Chris carefully, critically, placed every ornament, right down to each shimmering icicle, one at a time. My trees were a product of luck. Hers were a work of art.

For the first time, she had begun to show signs of the toll that battling three cancers over the past seven years had taken. Her face was drawn and she had developed stress lines. But she was still beautiful. Nothing could change that.

"You're prejudiced!" she said.

I had to admit that yes, I was.

Just as I also admired Chris for the way she had faced up

to her cancer, so did Don McIntyre. On a visit in the spring, he told her, "Except for your determination to live, there's no earthly reason why you're still alive.

"Just like your mother, you're a survival miracle!"

"My mother lived to be ninety-six," Chris said. "I don't think I'm going to be able to match that."

"Johan only had one cancer," Don reminded her. "You have three."

Dr. McIntyre no longer was in active practice. He still winged his white Jaguar in once a week and sat for a half-hour or so, chatting with Chris. Asking how she felt. Making helpful suggestions. I guess you're not a family doctor for fifty years without knowing a few things that some more recent members of the profession have yet to learn.

Chris's new primary physician was Maureen McConnell, of the Tuxedo Park Family Medical Centre, in Tuxedo Mall. Chris wanted her as a replacement for Dr. McIntyre. "There's not much chance Dr. McConnell will take me as a patient," Chris said. "Apparently she already has a full practice."

It is important for patients to have faith in their physicians. Perhaps this is particularly true for the chronically ill, like cancer patients. I figured that Maureen McConnell knew this as well as I did. I wrote her a page-long note about my wife. Some of it was her medical history. Most of it was about the gutsy way she had fought cancer for seven years. What it said basically was that Chris needed someone she could believe in.

Hippocrates taught that a good doctor's most important single trait is compassion. Maureen McConnell is a practising disciple. Her receptionist phoned Chris the next morning and set up her first appointment.

Chris's illness was becoming noticeably and more seriously progressive.

For the last couple of years, she had been taking Demerol for pain. This had been enough to hold her. Now she was on morphine twice daily, morning and evening. A visiting nurse, from the Victorian Order of Nurses, came by to do physical check-ups and treat for chronic, alternating bouts of diarrhea and bowel blockages.

Roanne, a professionally capable and personally caring person, became a regular visitor. It wasn't long before Chris began looking forward to her visits. It was apparent that Roanne enjoyed them, too.

After a while, Chris's kidney function began to fail. When she required daily aspirating to void, Roanne left the required equipment with me and showed me how to use it.

I already dispensed her morphine. We had begun this when I discovered that Chris repeatedly had forgotten that she already had medicated. Over a period of a half-hour or so, she had taken twice the prescribed amount. Roanne told me that this often happens when patients self-administer mind-altering drugs like morphine.

"At the very least it's dangerous," she said. "At the worst, sometimes fatal."

She advised me to put the morphine in a safe place—in effect to hide it—and to give it to Chris as prescribed. "When you're out of the house," Roanne said, "she might imagine that it's time for her medication and accidentally overdose. If she doesn't know where it is, this can't happen."

By fall, it became apparent that the "Grand Master," as Chris once had referred to her cancer, was moving towards checkmate. She had been getting a long-acting morphine that held her from morning through the day, and from evening through the night. It no longer did. Maureen McConnell prescribed a short-term morphine that Chris was required to take every four hours, twenty-four hours a day.

We usually went to bed at 10:00 p.m. I set the alarm for 2:00 a.m., got up, got the morphine from its hiding-place in the kitchen, and gave it to Chris with a glass of water. Then I set the alarm again for 6:00 a.m.: 10:00 a.m.: 2:00 p.m.: 6:00 p.m.: and to just before going back to bed, at 10:00 p.m.

Early on, as Chris switched off her bedside lamp, she joked "This reminds me of those nights when we had a new baby in the house. Sweet dreams!"

There can be unexpected and terrible consequences when just one link in the medical treatment chain snaps. We had dealt with a neighborhood pharmacy for years before and after Chris got cancer. We always had enjoyed a pleasant relationship.

When Chris's prescription was switched from delayed action to full release, four-hour morphine, the pharmacist did not catch the change. Whether through incompetence or carelessness, he went on filling the prescription with the same morphine as always.

Within a week, Chris began acting irrationally, sometimes violently, as though she had lost her mind. Afraid that she might injure herself, I phoned Maureen McConnell. She advised me to have her taken by ambulance to St. Boniface Hospital.

Dr. Jeff Sisler, of the Palliative Ward, had asked me to bring him Chris's medication. He checked the label and steered me into a meeting room. He held up the bottle. He looked very angry.

"Your wife's being poisoned by the wrong morphine," he said. "I checked with Dr. McConnell. She did not prescribe what you were given. I want you to switch to a pharmacy that knows something about drugs." He shoved the bottle into the pocket of his smock. "Then I suggest that you file a complaint against this druggist with the Manitoba Pharmaceutical Association."

I never did register a complaint. What was the point? The damage already had been done. I did refuse to pay the pharmacy for making my wife's last few months a worse hell than it otherwise would have been. The pharmacy later sued. I was advised to pay and countersue for malpractice. We settled out of court. I didn't countersue. Again I had to ask, What's the point? Every time he shaved, that pharmacist would have to look himself in the face. That was enough.

When she had recovered sufficiently, Chris came home. She was getting the proper medication, provided by a pharmacy across from St. Boniface Hospital. We were back on our four-hour medication breaks, but we could live with that. Chris was herself again.

We had a few good weeks together.

One of the most popular television series that fall was called "Thirtysomething." It was about a group of yuppies who worked for a Madison Avenue advertising agency. Everybody was well off, handsome, beautiful, clever, about to be named CEO, and searching both for Themselves and the Real Meaning of Life. Chris liked it because of her background in advertising.

The show's producers decided to have one of the wives get ovarian cancer. The disease strikes twenty thousand American women each year. Twelve thousand die from it. "Thirtysomething's" ratings hit an all-time high.

I did a quick channel switch when Nancy Weston, played by Patricia Wetig, was told she had ovarian cancer. I figured that Chris didn't need this.

"No," she said. "Let's watch."

It was curious. She listened and watched attentively, yet with an air of clinical detachment. It was as though she were witnessing her own dark passage into the world of "Nancy Weston," while at the same time examining the show for accuracy.

When the first episode was over, she said "It's good. Let's make a point of watching it." We did. Every week until Chris told me, one morning not long before Christmas, that she wanted to re-enter the Palliative Ward at St. Boniface Hospital.

Chris and I had talked often about how it should be when we reached this point.

She always had said that she wanted to die at home. I always had promised her that she would. Experiencing and learning about palliative care, during her recovery from wrongly dispensed drugs that had driven her berserk, had changed her mind.

"Those times I said I was scared," she explained, "I wasn't afraid of dying. I was afraid of the pain that comes with dying of cancer." She also told me bluntly that she did not want to be kept alive by what medical people call "heroic" means. "I don't want to be stuffed with tubes and have my breathing and heartbeat pumped up by machines. I want to be well," she said, "or I want to be dead."

She had given me a "living will" to this effect, which she had handwritten, dated and signed the previous year. I had recognized it for what it was: not an admission of defeat, but an act of preparation.

The word "palliative" means to make the patient comfortable without trying to cure the illness. The Palliative Ward at "St. B." does not allow the patient to die in pain. It has dual safeguards against this. One, referred to as "the ladder," escalates medication to the level required to keep the patient comfortable. The other, referred to as "the clock," ensures that it is repeated at precisely timed intervals, before the effects of the previous medication have worn off. No "heroic" means are used to keep the patient alive.

The care is individual. There are just twenty-eight beds in the ward. The doctors, nurses, and support staff all are special. It struck me that to be chosen for palliative care, they must undergo some sort of panning process whereby only the good-as-gold remain.

"Sometimes it must be very hard for them," Chris said. "They're always cheerful. Always there for us. You can tell that they really care. It must be very difficult for them when there are deaths in 'the family' month after month. I think it takes a certain kind of person to handle that."

There are no set visiting hours. I would arrive about noon every day with a "power shake" for Chris. We would go for a stroll, arm-in-arm, from her room up the corridor to a Common Room at the far end. It is furnished with a television set and comfortable chairs. There always is a fresh pot of coffee on, and hot water for tea. There is a large fridge where you can put perishable treats, like ice cream or cheese, with the patient's name on the package.

Families are encouraged to make the rooms as homelike as possible. I had furnished Chris's with some of her favorite things, including a photo with one of her father's sisters. It had been taken on a visit to the family croft, near Stornaway, in the Outer Hebrides. It had turned out very well, with the croft behind and the misty loch off in the distance. I took down another picture and hung it on the wall by her bed.

Chris had told the staff about Nigel. The head nurse suggested that I bring him in for a visit. The "personality kid" was a big hit. Whenever I figured Chris and he were getting lonesome for each other, I brought him back.

At about nine o'clock one evening, I phoned the ward and asked "May I say goodnight to my lady?" It became a ritual. "Everyone's come to expect your 'Goodnight, Lady' call," Chris laughed. "Every night, just before nine, someone goes for the plug-in phone!"

It was difficult to have favorites among the staff, but Jeff Sisler and a nurse we nicknamed "Irish" were extra special to both of us. Dr. Sisler was a complete professional. It was he who had spotted the improperly dispensed morphine that had made Chris so ill. Whenever we spoke with him about her condition, he was sensitive to our situation, but always up front with us. Both he and Maureen McConnell made us feel that we were all in this together.

We called our favorite nurse "Irish" because, as Chris put it, "She's such a colleen! She's young, pretty, and looks full of mischief. The minute she comes in the room, she makes me feel better."

A week or so before Christmas, Irish got Chris bundled up in a wheelchair to go shopping at Polo Park Mall. Chris enjoyed the festive feel of the place and revisiting all the familiar old stores and shops. We stopped to watch the children chatting with Santa. We bought gifts for our own grown children and the grandchildren.

I knew that the shopping trip had exhausted her. She surprised me, when we got back to the Palliative Ward, by suggesting that we have dinner together.

"I'll see if I can score an extra tray," I said.

"Oh, no! Not in my room. Not like I'm some sick person!" said Chris. "We're dining out tonight. Just like we used to!"

That worried me a little. I didn't think she was up to it.

But okay. I was game if she was. I wheeled the wheelchair around. "Where to?"

"There's a cozy little hideaway in the basement," said Chris.

We "dined out" in the hospital cafeteria. It was big and noisy. We managed to find an empty refectory table for ten that served as a table for two. I got plates for us both at the serving counter, looped a paper napkin over my arm, and played the waiter. It was just like old times. Almost.

A couple of days later, I walked into Chris's room with a table-top Christmas tree. Because it was artificial, she never would have let it into the house.

One thing Chris always did well was adjust to circumstances. She looked pleased when she saw the tree. I strung it with twinkle lights and decorated it with the little ornaments from "the bird tree." A few were originals, like the hand-crafted birds that gave the tree its name and that dated back to the early fifties. New to the tree were a Waterford crystal snowflake, bought while Chris was taking radiation in Calgary, and the tiny sailboat named *Carmel*.

I had asked Chris if she would like to celebrate Christmas by hosting a wine and cheese party for the Palliative Ward. She said yes. About noon on Christmas Eve, I arrived with a dozen or so different cheeses from aged Cheddar to Camembert. As many assorted kinds of crackers. Several bottles of Robert Mondavi red and white. A disposable Christmas tablecloth, plates, napkins, and wine glasses.

Irish wheeled a large metal table into Chris's room. It lost its institutional look under the bright red and green poinsettia tablecloth. She helped me lay out the wine and cheese buffet. I saw the bottles of wine get a couple of sidelong glances from passing staff.

"Am I breaking any rules?" I asked Irish.

"No one's ever done this before," she said, looking mischievous. "I don't think there *is* a rule. Yet."

The party went off beautifully. Staff, patients, and their visitors dropped in for the next hour or so and socialized over a cheese-plate and a glass of wine. It was all very Christmassy.

Chris played the hostess from her wheelchair. I could see that she was enjoying herself. Near the end, I gave her a Christmas Eve present. She sulked a little while she unwrapped it. "I wasn't able to get you anything," she said.

It was a boutique bottle of her trademark perfume, Shalimar by Guerlin, in a velvet box. It had been my gift to her on our first Christmas.

The card inside read *Dearest Christina: 41 years ago at Xmas I gave you this perfume because you love it and I loved you! I still love you, more than ever, and here again is Shalimar!*

Chris pressed my hand against her cheek. She gave Irish the card to read. "I think I'm going to cry," Irish said, meaning it.

Chris looked tired, but happy. The last of her guests were leaving, calling out their goodbyes. Chris responded with the closing lines of the traditional Christmas Eve poem.

"Merry Christmas to all," she said. "And to all a good night!"

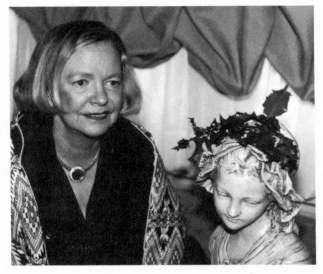

Christmas '90— For the first time, Chris began to show signs of the toll that battling three cancers over the past seven years had taken.

·Postscript

From the Winnipeg Free Press, Friday, January 31, 1992

An enduring cancer patient (never a victim!) with a remarkable sense of self died on Tuesday, January 28, in the Palliative Ward at St. Boniface General Hospital.

Christina (MacIver) Edge coexisted with colon and ovarian cancer and melanoma for eight years, through three major surgeries and one minor, chemotherapy, and radiation. Throughout these, she insisted on the patient's right to know and choose, deploring the arrogance of some doctors who she felt derogated and dehumanized patients.

She investigated and practised vitamin and visualization techniques promoted by Nobel Prize and other award-winning doctors and personally sought answers in Winnipeg, Toronto, Calgary, Vancouver, and San Francisco.

Through sheer determination and guts, she managed to live a good life for eight years, which, given her prognosis five or six years ago, upheld her personal philosophy that each person must take charge of their own life and that living well is the best revenge.

Christina was born in Winnipeg in 1928, the second daughter (the first predeceased in infancy) of Chief Constable Charles and Mrs. MacIver, both deceased. She attended St. Mary's Academy and United College, beginning a lengthy career in journalism and advertising as Assistant Women's Editor of *The Free Press*.

Married in 1950, she moved to Toronto and at various times lived in London, Paris, Malibu Beach, and Montreal. Returning to Winnipeg in 1967, she served as fashion writer, TV commercials producer, and special promotions director for the T. Eaton Co., Western Division, during which her work won various awards in New York and Chicago.

Christina is survived by her husband Fred; three sons, Rory, Casey and Shawn; a daughter, Elaine Osaka (Casey's wife) and two grandchildren, Tyson and Colin Osaka Edge; a brother, Don MacIver; and a loyal and little friend, Nigel, a King Charles Spaniel. Another brother, Charles MacIver, predeceased her.

Special mention must be make of the following: Dr. Don McIntyre, who was Christina's primary physician for many years and remained her personal friend, regular weekly visitor, and medical confidante right up to her admittance to the Palliative Ward; Dr. Maureen McConnell, of the Tuxedo Park Family Medical Centre, who well represents the new breed of honest, no-nonsense doctors and latterly was her primary physician; and Dr. Jeff Sisler, of the Palliative Ward, who also qualifies both on the grounds of unquestionable competence and the patient's need and right to know.

Not enough can be said of the nurses and support staff of the Palliative Ward. These are the Angels in White who transcend the popular notion of today's medical service people. They do the special extra. They provide the personal and professional love and care that make it possible to leave the dying beloved in someone else's caring hands. Bless them all for this.

As a hobby, Christina bred and showed Standard Poodles under the Canadian Kennel Club registration Bucko Kennels. Those wishing to do something nice for her might consider a donation to the Winnipeg Humane Society.

She was cremated. She and her husband will unite once more in a celebration of life in the Cathedral of the Rockies.

On the morning of March 9, son Shawn and I, accompanied by Nigel, deposited Chris's ashes at the far end of the lake, at the base of the mountain, in that part of the Rockies that she loved best.

I said these words: "Dear Friend, Wife and Mother—If there is a God, you will go to him Godspeed from here. If life is like the oceans and the mountains, then you are safe now in the arms of Mother Earth. Rest in beauty and in peace, my love. You have earned it."

•Referrals

At the beginning of *Borrowed Time*, I noted that this is not a medical book. I advised readers with cancer to consult with a medical professional. To learn personally all they could about their disease. Perhaps to consider alternative therapies as a complement to conventional medicine, as Chris did. Then to make their own informed decisions.

The same advice applies to Referrals.

There are a thousand and one books out there on cancer. Many of them promise everything from how never to get cancer to a "miracle cure" if you do. The following nine books and four services were chosen because each comes with strong credentials. Chris and I found them to be a great help in our better understanding of cancer and her decisions on how to combat it.

Since we all differ in our psychological, physiological, and physical makeups, the advice and programs in one or another of these books or services may not be right for you.

Before making any decisions on conventional medical treatment and alternative therapies, particularly diet or vitamin programs, as described both in *Borrowed Time* and

Referrals, talk to a doctor who is both knowledgeable and willing to discuss them with you.

CONVENTIONAL MEDICINE

Choices: Realistic Alternatives in Cancer Treatment.
Marion Morra and Eve Potts.
Avon Books
105 Madison Avenue, New York, N.Y. 10016

Chris used to call her dog-eared copy of *Choices* "the only book on conventional cancer treatment that anyone really needs." (While the subtitle uses the term "Alternatives," the reference is to medical alternatives, not alternative therapies.) Written in a comprehensive question-and-answer format, it covers all of the common types of cancer from symptoms through staging and treatment. It also deals with side effects and many of the psychological and physical aspects of living with cancer.

Drugs Used in Conventional Medicine

PDR Family Guide to Prescription Drugs.
Medical Economics Data,
5 Paragon Drive, Montvale, New Jersey 07645

One of the first steps in becoming an active partner in your own health care is knowing what is being done to you and why. This includes what drugs you are being given. The *PDR Family Guide to Prescription Drugs* has overviews on all of the chronic diseases, such as heart disease and arthritis, as well as cancer. It indexes drugs, detailing why they were prescribed, how and when they should be taken, and possible side effects.

ALTERNATIVE THERAPIES

Acupuncture

Thorsons Introductory Guide to Acupuncture.
Paul Marcus, M.D.
Thorsons - Harper Collins
77 - 85 Fulham Place Road
Hammersmith, London, W68JB

Dr. Marcus frankly admits that neither he nor anyone else knows why acupuncture works. He qualifies this with the observation that acupuncture is not alone among medical treatments that work without science knowing why. He also points out that acupuncture has an impressive track record. It has been practised in China for some 5,000 years. It increasingly is being acknowledged, particularly in the area of chronic pain control, in the West. This book answers all of the basic questions about acupuncture, from its ancient origins to what it might be able to accomplish for you. Marcus also gives case histories.

Diet and Nutrition

Nutritional Therapy:
Featuring the Core Program for Diet Revision
Stephen Gilason, M.D.
Persona Publications
1 - 3661 West Fourth Avenue
Vancouver, B.C. V6R 1P2

Most doctors are not knowledgeable about nutrition. When Chris asked about it, she usually got the reply "Eat sensibly." To which she invariably asked herself (and me) "Eat what sensibly?" Dr. Gilason calls his Core Program "human software" and suggests that it be modified to suit the individual. It is not a weight control diet, though he suggests this may be a bonus. It is intended to help prevent or control chronic diseases. The book deals with the pathology of body-food interactions, considers the dangers of contaminants, pesticides and many food additives, and lists healthy food choices, with preparation and menu planning.

Therapeutic Touch

Therapeutic Touch: A Practical Guide.
Janet Macrae.
Alfred Knopf Inc.
201 East 50th Street, New York, N.Y. 10022

Therapeutic touch is another ancient form of healing that until relatively recently was dismissed as hocus-pocus by most doctors, and still is by many. Practised for centuries in Europe, the technique was pioneered in the United States by Dora Kunz. Dolores Krieger, Ph.D. Nursing, also became convinced that therapeutic touch worked. They developed the "Krieger-Kunz Model of Therapeutic Touch," based on research by Kunz, Krieger, and others over four years at centres in the United States and Canada, including Montreal's prestigious McGill University. In 1975, Krieger began a class in "TT" at New York University. Nurse-members of that first class, and those that followed, became apostles. Throughout North America, therapeutic touch has mushroomed since. Macrae's book explains in simple terms the origin of its modern revival and how and why it works.

Visualization

Getting Well Again.
O. Carl Simonton M.D., D.A.B.R.
with Stephanie Matthews-Simonton
and James L. Creighton.
Bantam Books, Inc.
666 Fifth Avenue, New York, N.Y. 10103

Husband-and-wife Carl and Stephanie Simonton are recognized internationally as leaders in the field of holistic health care. In hospitals throughout the United States, they have established cancer counselling programs modelled on their own Cancer Counselling and Research Center, in Dallas, Texas. This book examines the link between stress and illness. It provides self-help ways to a positive attitude, pain management, goal setting, and detailed visualization techniques. It also details exercise programs for patients in all stages of cancer and how to establish a family support system.

Love, Medicine and Miracles:
Lessons Learned about Self-Healing
from a Surgeon's Experience with Exceptional Patients
Bernard Siegel, M.D.
Harper and Row, Publishers
10 East 53rd. Street, New York, N.Y. 10022.

In many ways, this is much like the Simontons' book. It deals with the relationship between cancer (or any chronic disease) and the mind. Dr. Siegel explains his faith in the power of "the will to live," backed up by his many years of experience with cancer patients and supported by case histories. He guides the reader through visualization. He explains why "bad" patients tend to live longer than "good" ones. Clearly, Siegel is a medical professional who believes in "love and miracles" at least as much as he does in conventional medicine.

Vitamins

Cancer and Vitamin C:
A Discussion of the Nature, Causes, Prevention
and Treatment of Cancer,
with Special Reference to the Value of Vitamin C
Linus Pauling, Ph.D.,
Nobel Chemistry and Peace Prizes
with Ewan Cameron, M.D., Ch.B.
F.R.C.S. Glasgow and Edinburgh.
Camino Books Inc.
PO Box 59026, Philadelphia, PA. 19102

Millions of people world-wide take Vitamin C to strengthen their immune system against the common cold. The basic premise for this book is that Vitamin C also can work to prevent cancer or to prolong the life of the cancer patient. The book examines the values and limitations of both conventional medical and unconventional treatment. Its conclusions, drawn from case histories and clinical trials, have been the subject of ongoing controversy for years. Each side—those who support Vitamin C therapy and those who don't—claims the other's findings are flawed. The book tells how to self-administer Vitamin C as therapy. It also examines foods, nutrition, and the value of other vitamins and minerals.

Dr. Moerman's Anti-Cancer Diet:
Holland's Revolutionary Program for Combatting Cancer.
Ruth Jochems.
Avery Publishing Group Inc.
Garden City Park, New York

Although this book has "Diet" in its title, it properly belongs under "Vitamins." Dr. Moerman's anti-cancer program is based on eight vitamins and minerals that are taken daily to supplement those found naturally in the foods recommended in his diet. Moerman began research into anti-cancer nutrition in the 1930s and was ridiculed for years by the Dutch medical establishment. Vindiction came in 1987, when independent clinical trials led the government of The Netherlands to declare the Moerman Diet effective in cancer prevention and treatment. *Dr. Moerman's Anti-Cancer Diet* was written by Ruth Jochems, who, after his sister was diagnosed with cancer, became a disciple of Moerman and collaborated with him on the book. Jochems tells us how the vitamins and minerals should be taken and why they work. He gives Spartan menus and recipes. Not for the uncommitted!

PERSONAL SERVICES

Diet and Nutrition

Provincial Dietetic Associations

Patients who prefer a one-on-one approach to establishing their personal diet program should consult with a trained and registered professional. Members of provincial dietetic associations have a university degree in foods and nutrition, followed by a year's in-hospital or community experience. Look for the provincial name in the white pages of your telephone book, or in the yellow pages under "Dieticians and Nutritionists." Registered practitioners have the initials "CDA" after their name.

Medical Updates

Planetree Health Resource Center
2040 Webster Street, San Francisco, CA 94115
Phone 415-923-3681.

Planetree began as a non-profit medical library in 1981. It was established to provide the public with state-of-the-art information on medical diagnoses, experimental and conventional procedures, and prognoses. In response to demand from outside San Francisco, it soon escalated to a mail service. For patients who wish to be informed about their disease and its treatment, Planetree provides a choice of three packages. The first is the one that Chris found so useful. "In-Depth" consists of updates on conventional and alternative treatments; selections from current medical texts, journals and consumer health literature; and bibliography ($100). "Bibliography" provides summaries of current articles and a computerized search of source-books from the database of the U.S. National Library of Medicine ($35). "Basic Packet" is a compilation of current, general information on symptoms, treatment, and prognosis ($20). Phone or write for brochure or to order. Cheque, Visa, or MasterCard. Fees are in $ U.S.

Therapeutic Touch

Nurse Healers—Professional Associates Inc.
PO Box 444, Allison Park, Penn., 15101
Phone 412-355-8476.

Although there are some 10,000 registered practitioners of therapeutic touch in Canada and the United States, and thousands more in over thirty-six other countries worldwide, they are just now (1995) beginning to organize. In Canada, Ontario and Alberta are the only two provinces that have formed therapeutic touch associations. Others are in the process. Anyone outside Ontario and Alberta wishing to contact a registered practitioner in his or her area should phone or write the association listed above.

Visualization

Hope Cancer Health Centre
2574 West Broadway Avenue, Vancouver, B.C. V6K 2G1
Phone 604-732-3412

Hope is a non-profit, cancer patient and family support group that was begun by cancer patient Claude Dosdall in 1980. Staff, all of whom have been diagnosed with cancer, provide monthly group therapy and visualization workshops, periodic retreats, and ongoing individual and family counselling, in person or by phone. The Centre's programs are meant to complement conventional medical treatment. Their objective not only is to help patients and their families to learn to live with cancer, but also to show them how to get the most out of life in the process. Phone counselling is available from 10:00 a.m. to 4:00 p.m., Monday through Friday. Phone or write for brochure, application for weekend workshops, and newsletter. Tax-deductible donations welcomed.

Index

Senokot, 17.
Tagamet, 53.
Tylenol 3, 44.
Valium, 24, 25.
Drugs, high tolerance for, 25.
Drugs, side effects, 53, 100,
116, 120, 123, 126.

Power shakes, 127, 175, 179, 183, 216.
Prepping for procedures:
Self-prep, 15, 17, 23.
Hospital prep, 29, 97.
Prince Charles, 149.
Private nurse, 93, 104.
Pruden, Gordon and Eileen, 206.

· Q

Quality of life, 109, 114, 133.
Quebec shillelagh, 42, 45, 58, 82, 114.
Queen Elizabeth, 149, 159.
Queen Mother, 79, 149.

· R

Radiation side effects, 170, 178, 183, 187.
Radiation simulator, 178.
Radner, Gilda, 16, 205.
Ramona island cottage, 74, 113, 156, 185.
Reagan, U.S. President Ronald and Nancy, 149.
Recovery room, 32, 93, 105.
Respiratory arrest, 20, 88.
Ross, Dr. Charlotte, 29, 47, 70.

· S

Sister Mary Anne, 94, 99, 104.
Spousal:
Care-giving, 194, 212.
Feelings of guilt, 124, 209.
Honesty, 86, 96.
Need to communicate, 57, 199.

Overprotectiveness, 48, 198.
Sense of Rejection, 126.
Supportiveness, 17, 23, 36, 73, 91, 104, 117, 134, 183.
Stoma (see Colostomy)
Sun-lamps, 185.
Surgical procedures:
Appendectomy, 106.
Biopsy, 13, 24, 34, 73, 185.
Colostomy, 28, 33, 34.
Exploratory, 208.
Hysterectomy, 106, 108.
Laparotomy (see Exploratory)
Mastectomy, 180.
Omentectomy, 106.
Sigmoid colon resection, 16, 34.
Survivalists, 198.

· T

T-cells (see Immune system)
Tea ladies (see Tom Baker Cancer Centre)
Terminal patients, 16.
Tom Baker Cancer Centre (see Hospitals and clinics)
"Thirtysomething," the TV series, 214.
TT (See Alternative therapies: Therapeutic Touch)
Tumors:
Benign, 13, 25.
Malignant, 13, 16, 26, 34.
Tuxedo Villa, Winnipeg, 30, 82.

· U

United College, Winnipeg (see

below)
University of Winnipeg, 49, 92.

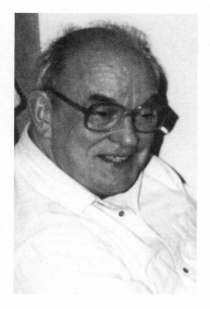

Fred Edge has been a reporter, editor, and award-winning columnist for major daily newspapers and has published more than 200 magazine articles. His television series and anthology dramas have been seen on Canadian and American network television. His first book was *Don't Tell Me About It, Write It!—How to get and write the news for newspapers*, (The Press Journal, Toronto, 1967). His second was the biography of Charlotte Whitehead Ross, one of Canada's first woman doctors. *The Iron Rose*, published in 1992 by the University of Manitoba Press, led the Manitoba government, in 1993, to legislate Charlotte Ross the right to practise medicine, 77 years after her death. As a young man, Fred Edge abandoned his own plans to study medicine when he left pre-med at the University of Ottawa and joined the newsroom staff of the *Ottawa Citizen*. He now lives in Victoria, BC.